PEGAN D

333 Quick and Easy Recipes to Burn Fat and Jumpstart losing weight by combining Keto, Paleo, and Vegan Diets all in one! 31-Day Food Journal Included.

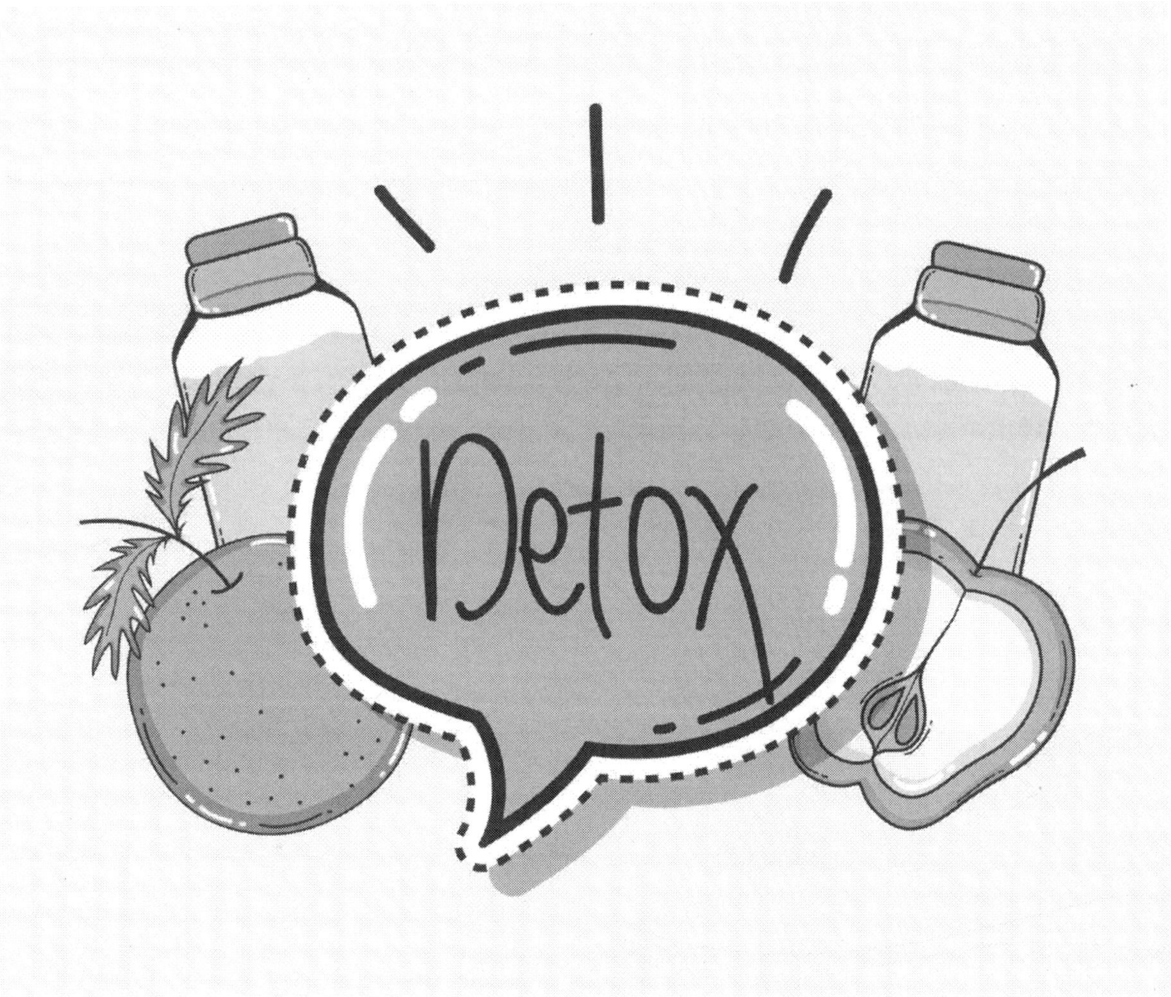

![Detox illustration]

Contents

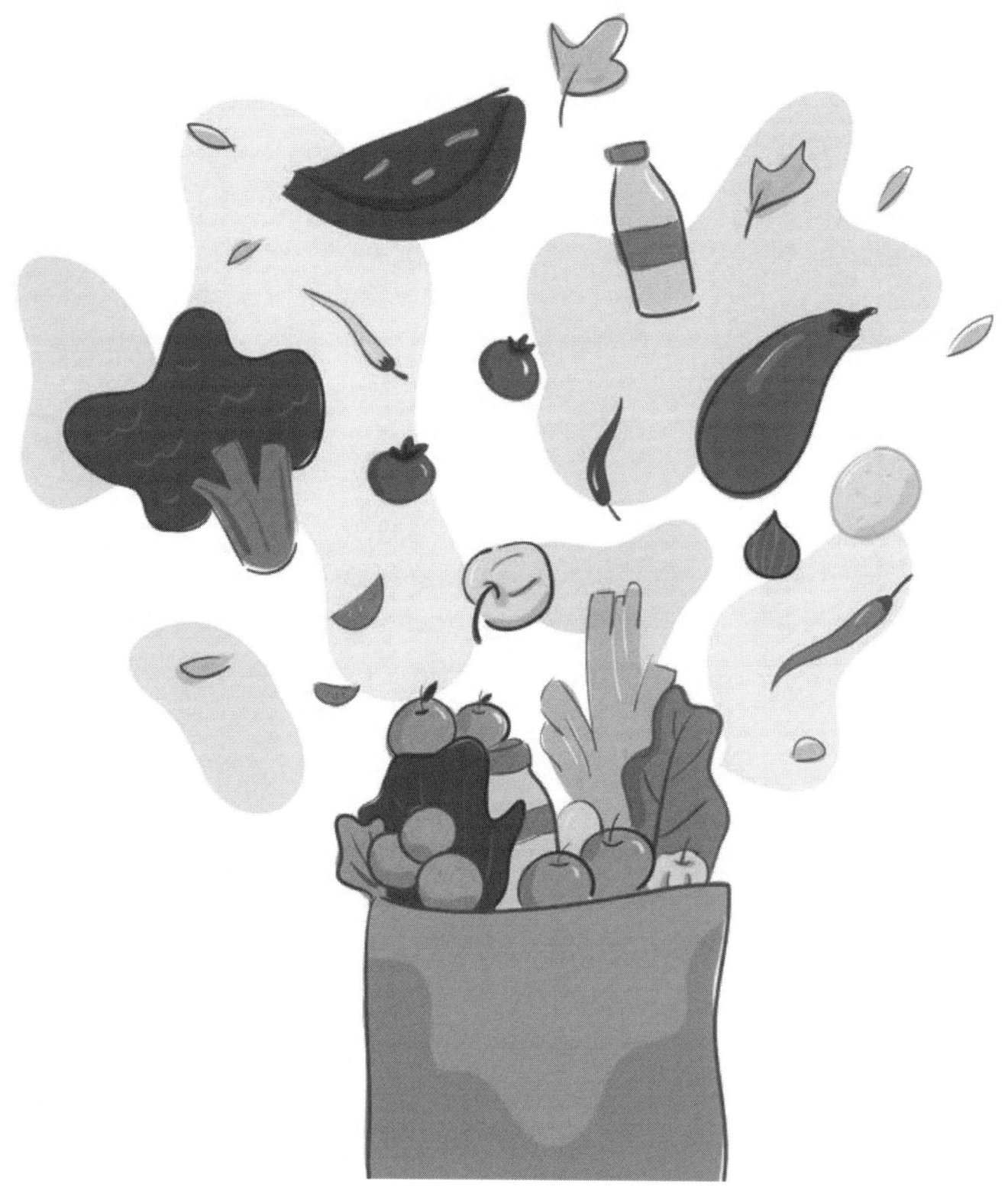

Chapter 1: Introduction to Pegan Diet

What is Pegan Diet

The Pegan diet joins a few paleo diets and veganism standards and recommends a plant-principally based eating vogue. Devotees eat vegetables, natural products, nuts, seeds, meat, fish, and eggs and keep away from dairy, grains, vegetables, sugar, and handled nourishments. Its limitation can construct the Pegan diet rigid to continue over the long haul. Ice the name recommends the Pegan diet acquires standards from each the paleo diet and veganism. So, paleo eaters endeavor to devour exclusively food sources offered inside the Paleolithic period 2.6 million years prior: vegetables, organic products, nuts, fish, and meat. It regularly avoids dairy, grains, sugar, vegetables, oils, salt, liquor, and low. Veganism endorses avoiding any creature items and side-effects - along with meat, fish, eggs, cheddar, yoghurt, and nectar - and eating plant-fundamentally based nourishments all things considered. The Pegan diet consolidates basic standards from paleo, and veggie lover eats less principally dependent on the idea that supplement thick, whole food sources can decrease aggravation, balance glucose, and backing ideal well-being. If your first idea is that going paleo and veggie lover all the while sounds almost unthinkable, you are in good company. Notwithstanding its name, the Pegan diet is unmistakable and has its arrangement of rules. In all actuality, it is less prohibitive than either a paleo or veggie lover diet without help from anyone else. Significant accentuation is set on vegetables and natural product. However, little to direct meat, sure fish, nuts, seeds, and a couple of vegetables is also permitted. Vigorously prepared sugars, oils, and grains are debilitated - anyway still adequate in tiny sums. The Pegan diet isn't planned as a standard, transient eating routine. All things being equal, it plans to be a ton of practical along these lines that you will follow it inconclusively. The Pegan diet is predicated on paleo and veggie lover standards - however, it empowers some meat utilization. It stresses entire nourishments, particularly vegetables, while to a great extent disallowing gluten, dairy, most grains, and vegetables. It is wealthy in a few supplements that may advance ideal well-being anyway might be excessively prohibitive for some individuals. You can give this eating regimen an endeavor to decide how your body reacts. In case you are as of now paleo or vegetarian and are curious about changing your eating regimen, the Pegan diet may be simpler to acclimate to. The paleo diet is intended to look like what human agrarian progenitors ate millennia back. Even though it is difficult to decisively get a handle on what human predecessors ate in a few pieces of the planet, scientists accept their eating regimens comprised of entire nourishments. By following an entire food-basically based eating regimen and driving dynamic lives, tracker finders had plentiful lower paces of the way of life illnesses, for example, corpulence, diabetes and coronary disease. Indeed, a few examinations prescribe that this eating routine can prompt critical weight reduction (while not calorie checking) and significant upgrades in well-being. Both the paleo and veggie lover eat fewer cars are at the center of attention as of late for their independent ways to deal with food and well-being. Many people on the whole likelihood expect them as total inverses, with paleo that work in meats our predecessors hypothetically ate and veganism quitting creature item by and large. Notwithstanding, a relatively new gobbling set up means to show that meat-genuine paleo and veggie-driven veganism will coincide in a solitary eating routine. The Pegan diet (as in, paleo + veggie lover), made by superstar deliberate medication specialist Mark Hyman, M.D., indicates to offer the most astonishing aspect of every universe. The eating routine educates filling 75% regarding your plate with plant-based generally nourishments and twenty-five% with lean, economically raised meats. As per Dr Hyman, eating this implies can scale back the peril of persistent sickness, control irritation, and advance general well-being. Paleo consumes fewer calories seem to attempt to do something very similar. Since its beginning in 2014, the Pegan diet has consistently acquired consideration among those needing for tips for clean good dieting. In contrast to specific eating regimens, agnosticism doesn't give rules for explicitly what to have for breakfast, lunch, and supper. Or maybe, it gives an overall blueprint of dietary guidance dependent on various essential standards. The great fundamentals of a Pegan diet embrace picking nourishments with an espresso glycemic load; eating heaps of natural products, vegetables, nuts, and seeds (concerning 3/4 of your everyday admission), picking grass-took care of or economically raised meats when you do eat meat; staying away from synthetic substances, added substances, pesticides, and GMOs; acquiring bunches of sound fats like omega-3s and unsaturated fat; and eating naturally and territorially. Since the Pegan diet advances a general example of eating, it doesn't offer rules around the circumstance of dinners or snacks-nor does it give suggestions on how a great deal of to eat in a very day, or which segment sizes to pick. You will not be expected to dominate a specific cooking strategy or buy particular items, though on a Pegan diet. Because the arrangement is still similarly new, assets on an approach to follow aren't pretty much as broadly reachable as a few distinctive, elegant eating plans. In any case, as premium in the eating regimen has risen, increasingly more Pegan cookbooks (and even a modest bunch of food stock, as Pegan protein bars) have hit the market. Your smartest choice for discovering assets on clinging to the Pegan diet is doubtlessly the net, where blog entries and sites give plans that follow the entire nourishments, 3-quarter-plants, and one-quarter meat rules. The Pegan diet is quite possibly the latest patterns to arise in the well-being scene. This veggie lover diet- paleo diet crossover gobbling set up guarantees sharp weight reduction, better glucose the board and diminished aggravation, with huge loads of Pegan diet audits available web-based hailing its simplicity and viability. On the contrary, the eating regimen is hard to follow, inadequate and superfluously prohibitive. Nowadays, it seems like everybody is talking concerning the Pegan diet - the low-starch, moderate protein, high-fat eating plan that changes your body into a fat-consuming machine. Hollywood stars and expert competitors have openly promoted this current eating regimens advantages, from getting in shape, bringing down glucose, battling aggravation, lessening malignancy hazard, expanding energy, to hindering maturing. Consequently, is Pegan one thing that you should consider dominating? The accompanying can present a defense for what this eating routine is concerning, the experts and cons, notwithstanding the issues to show up out for. Regularly, the body utilizes glucose as the most stockpile of fuel for energy. At the point when you are on a Pegan diet, and you are eating extremely not many carbs with just moderate measures of protein (abundance protein can be changed over to carbs), your body switches its fuel supply to run generally on fat. The liver produces muscles (a sort of unsaturated fat) from fat. These muscles become a fuel supply for the body, particularly the cerebrum which devours masses of energy and can run on one or the other glucose or muscles. At the point when the body produces muscles, it enters a metabolic state alluded to as Pegan. Fasting is the easiest way to accomplish Pegan. At the point when you are fasting or eating not many carbs and just moderate measures of protein, your body goes to consuming put away fat for fuel. That is the reason people will, in general, lose extra weight on the Pegan diet. You need to recall that the body utilizes sugar, looking like glycogen to work. The Pegan diet that is exceptionally limited in sugar powers your body to utilize fat as fuel instead of sugar, since it doesn't get sufficient sugar. When the body doesn't get sufficient sugar for fuel, the liver is compelled to transform the out of their fat into muscles used by the body as fuel - thus the term Pegan. This eating regimen could be a high-fat eating routine with reasonable measures of protein. Contingent upon your carb admission the body arrives at a province of Pegan in yet each week and stays there. As fat is utilized instead of sugar for fuel inside the body, the weight misfortune is sensational while no alleged limitation of calories. The Pegan diet is with the end goal that you should mean to instigate sixty-75percent of your day-by-day calories from fat, fifteen-thirty from protein and just five-10p.c from starches. This regularly implies that you can eat just 20-fifty grams of carbs in an extremely day. For a few people, the Pegan diet could be an extraordinary opportunity for weight reduction. It is entirely unexpected and licenses the individual on the eating routine to eat an eating regimen that comprises food sources that you may not anticipate. In this way, the Pegan diet, or Pegan, could be an eating routine that comprises exceptionally low carbs and high fat. How a few weight control plans are there where you can start your downtime with bacon and eggs, heaps of it, and follow it up with chicken wings for lunch and steak and broccoli for supper. That may sound unrealistic for some. This eating regimen is regularly an incredible day of eating, and you followed the establishments consummately with that feast set up. When you eat a low amount of carbs, your body gets place into a territory of Pegan. What this proposes is your body consumes fat for energy. How low of a measure of carbs do you wish to eat to instigate into Pegan? Indeed, it shifts from individual to individual. Anyway, it is a sure thing to remain under 25 net carbs. A few would propose that when no doubt about its acceptance is the point at which you are truly placing your body into Pegan, you should keep underneath ten net carbs. On the off chance that you don't know what net carbs are, let me encourage you. Web carbs are the number of carbs you eat short the amount of dietary fiber. Along these lines, if you eat a sum of 35 grams of web carbs and thirteen grams of dietary fiber, your net carbs for the day would be 22. Sufficiently simple, isn't that so? All in all, other than weight reduction, what else is sweet about Pegan? Numerous people talk concerning their improved mental clearness on when on the eating regimen. Another benefit has an ascent in energy. One more is a diminished craving. One factor to worry over when happening the Pegan diet is something many refer to as Pegan influenza. Not every person encounters this, aside from this that do it tends to be intense. You can feel torpid, and you may have a migraine. It won't keep going exceptionally long. When you are feeling this way verify you get masses of water and rest to initiate through it. On the off chance that this seems as though the sort of diet you would be interested about, at that point, what are you anticipating? Jump heard first into Pegan. You won't accept the outcomes you get in a concise amount of time.

Basics of Pegan Diet

Have you needed to instigate that physical make-up anyway felt that you needed to lose some weight first? Or then again could it be that the expression "weight reduction"; has been sticking around in the back of your psyche, simply that you just never very got down to dealing with it? Prohibitive and peculiar eating regimens, costly whimsical machines, and the last fat-consuming, no- exercise wizardry weight reduction pill. This future, the different implied arrangements that one would see at whatever point you request an answer inside the astonishing, multi-billion-dollar weight reduction exchange. In all actuality, by getting back to the current book, you have just got a suspicion of what is truly expected to impact protected and enduring weight reduction.

- It is a characteristic truth that exclusively through watching what we eat, will we generally affect our weight. This is the place where the Pegan diet very sparkles and empowers you to savor programmed, simple fat-consuming without all the standard calorie limitations of various eating regimens. Weight reduction is a sure outcome you will appreciate once you start the Pegan diet, anyway this can be not the only advantage you will get delighted from.
- Think about every one of those exercises you have continually wished to seek after yet racked because you essentially had no energy left once your normal days' worth of effort. The chance to mud off those pastimes and subsequently the stuff you relish doing, because of the Pegan diet, will have more energy for your day-by-day work and play! The going with mental clearness and sharpness of thought additionally are constructive outcomes that you will have as an immediate consequence of the eating regimen.
- A higher well-being report card, by methods for enhanced cholesterol readings, standardized glucose and a comparing brought down danger of cardiovascular sicknesses likewise are just a portion of the beneficial well-being impacts experienced by most on the eating routine. This current book is point is principally to control the devices with which to allow the Pegan to slim down run all the more easily and flawlessly in your lifestyle.
- Many learn that an eating routine is exclusively as slick as the number of plans it is in its collection. The advantages of an express eating routine may be changed, however on the off chance that you are compelled to claim similar stuff each morning meal, lunch and supper, even the most devoted ally of the part would doubtlessly have issues supporting the eating regimen. This is frequently where I am generally glad to refer to that the Pegan diet has very some elbow room for the creation of different entirely unexpected plans, and it is the reason for this book to present to you a portion of the more heavenly and easy-to-get ready dinners for your gastronomic delight!
- For the fledglings still, because the Pegan diet is adepts, the plans contained inside are made explicitly to be hitting home with your sense of taste while not expecting you to in a real sense pay the whole day inside the kitchen! Succinct and forthright, the plans separate feast arrangement needs during a direct evaluation by grade design, simple for anybody to see.

- An additional multi-day feast set up is organized to serve each steerage with motivation for the new and ongoing disciples to the Pegan diet. Staple records prime everything off to introduce you the opportune update on what to get on your next food shopping trip. The very truth you are here with this book is adequate evidence that you are at least curious to see how the Pegan diet can help you. Significantly higher, perhaps you are as of now very knowledgeable with its advantages and are looking for assorted, rich, and grandiose plans for a multi-day part of delightful Pegan venture.

- Notwithstanding that this Pegan diet cookbook can be very much positioned to furnish you with significant culinary thoughts to support your day-by-day dinners. I expect that the value and thoughts you find in this book can work well for you, and might you have a productive Pegan venture! The Pegan diet is all about new, healthy nourishments, delighted in offset with each unique and what your body normally wants. Nutritionists consistently illuminate gobble the rainbow by stacking up on ongoing vegetables and natural products, and that is sound counsel. When you receive a Pegan attitude, you might have the option to work out what is best for you.

- Plants-and a wide reach at that-offer us with vast energy and the vita-minutes and minerals we tend to have to fuel our days. The Pegan diet urges us to make suppers included 75 % new and, preferably, pesticide-5 produce. This recommendation is additionally a 100 % disrupter of how a few depict the standard American eating regimen. A 4-to six-ounce part of meat or fish works best, furnishing us with indispensable nutrients and minerals, for example, I3, a couple of, iron, potassium, zinc, and phosphorus, that are troublesome or impractical to ask from a veggie lover diet. Grass-took care of meat likewise contains formed linoleic acids, which encourage with fat misfortune, fit muscle advancement, and diabetes avoidance.

- These acids even have cancer prevention agents like beta carotene and nutrient K. Economically made meat, fish, and eggs conjointly have a more modest carbon impression, squeezing the climate overall. Contingent upon where you live. It is likewise helpful to eat an extra plant-fundamentally based eating regimen utilizing occasional fixings. There might be a motivation behind why we will, in general, want brilliant green vegetables after an extended, cold winter; lighter, better vegetables inside the late spring when the mercury rises: and heartier produce as the climate cools in pre-winter, especially as we incline tore needing extra food to support the – resting; to come. Our bodies are mentioning to us what we need what is more, when.

- Accordingly, momentarily, eating an eating regimen comprising predominantly of plants with some meat, fish and omega-3 rich eggs-guarantees you may get all the supplements along with protein, you wish not simply to work, anyway live, and live well.

What do you eat on the Pegan diet?
The essential nutritional category for the Pegan diet is vegetables and organic product – this thought is to contain 75 per cent of your unlimited admission. Low-glycemic leafy foods, similar to berries and non-bland vegetables, should be accentuated to weaken your glucose reaction. Small measures of bland vegetables and sweet organic products could be considered individuals who have just accomplished reliable glucose control past to starting the eating routine. Albeit the Pegan diet fundamentally accentuates plant food sources, satisfactory protein admission from creature sources stays propelled. Remember that since seventy, this should of the eating regimen comprises vegetables and organic product, under 25% remaining parts for creature-based proteins. You will have a 25 piece of lower meat admission than you would on a standard paleo diet – anyway still extra than on any vegetarian diet. The Pegan diet debilitates eating traditionally cultivated meats or eggs. All things being equal, it places weight on grass-took care of, field raised wellsprings of meat, pork, poultry, and entire eggs. Furthermore, it energizes fish admission - explicitly individuals who keep an eye on own low mercury content super tight and wild salmon. As anyone might expect, meat contains the paleo part of going Pegan. The eating routine stresses picking meats like hamburger, chicken, and sheep and other, extra remarkable ones like ostrich or buffalo that are grass-taken care of, economically raised, and privately sourced. Nonetheless, note that meat makes up exclusively a minority of the food you will eat on a Pegan diet, what is more, presently for the vegetarian feature of things! Most of the calories on a Pegan diet

come from plant-based generally food sources like soil products. Not at all like Paleo is standards about those organic products or vegetable cave dwellers would have eaten, Paganism doesn't separate. All assortments of turn out are permitted on the eating routine however Hyman energizes choosing ones with low glycemic load, similar to berries or watermelon, when possible. Nuts and seeds give other fiber, protein, and micronutrients on a Pegan diet. They are furthermore a wellspring of good monounsaturated and omega-3 fats. Gags are another proper protein for agnostics. This morning meal food exemplary gives nutrient B12, which may run low during a restricted meat diet. A few contrasts between paleo versus vegetarian eat fewer carbs, which can construct it trying to aggregate a Pegan diet looking through rundown that joins each component. The eating routine spotlights entire, natural food sources with heaps of soil products to a great extent. Dissimilar to the antiquated paleo diet, modest quantities of grains and vegetables are allowed, for example, quinoa, oats, beans and chickpeas. Nonetheless, admission should be limited to not more than a 0.5 cup of grains each day and yet one cup of vegetables. Economically sourced meat, poultry, fish and eggs are permitted on the eating routine with some restraint. This incorporates food sources like wild-got fish, free-differ poultry and grass-took care of hamburger. This is impressively entirely unexpected than ordinary vegetarian eats fewer carbs, that wipes out all creature-based product from the eating routine. Even though fish isn't the star of a Pegan diet is, it puts in this eating organize. Hyman states that low-mercury fish super tight, herring, and anchovies are satisfactory fish.

- Fish: Select choices with low mercury, such as sardines, herring and anchovies.
- Meat: The focus on grass-fed beef, pork and poultry are on.
- Eggs: Eggs are an inexpensive source of nutrients and protein that are important.
- Soft drinks, fruit juices, table sugar, sweets, pastries, ice cream and many more. Sugar and high-fructose corn syrup:
- Vegetables: The rest of the diet is low-glycemic (non-starchy) vegetables.
- Fruit: the higher the variety, the better the
- Nuts: Besides peanuts, eat plenty of almonds, pistachios, walnuts, and other nuts.
- Seeds: The thumbs-up is also offered to flax, chia, pumpkin, and other seeds.
- Grains: Bread and pasta, wheat, spelt, rye, barley, etc. included.
- Legumes: Lentils, beans and many more.
- Dairy: Avoid most dairy products, especially low-fat ones (include full-fat dairies like butter and cheese).
- The following vegetable oils are used: soybean oil, sunflower oil, cottonseed oil, corn oil, grape oil, safflower oil, etc.
- Trans fats: discovered in margarine and different processed foods. Typically referred to as oils that are hydrogenated or partly hydrogenated.
- Artificial sweeteners: aspartame, sucralose, potassium acesulfame, cyclamate, saccharin. Instead, using natural sweeteners.
- Highly processed foods: Everything labelled diet or low-fat or that has many additives. Includes artificial meal replacements.

Foods to Avoid in Pegan Diet

The Pegan diet is extra adaptable than a paleo or vegetarian diet since it permits regular admission of pretty much any food. A few food sources and food groups are debilitated. A portion of those nourishments is known to be undesirable, while others may be considered exceptionally sound - relying upon whom you inquire. Set aside the pizza and frozen yoghurt, you won't eat dairy on a Pegan diet. Hyman accepts cow is milk adds to corpulence, coronary illness, diabetes, and malignant growth. Following the paleo reasoning, agnosticism disregards practically all grains.

Consequently wheat, oats, grain, bulgur, and a few others will not show up on a Pegan plate. The hypothesis goes that grains increment glucose and can cause aggravation. Restricted utilization of bound low-glycemic grains is at times worthy on the eating regimen, similar to a 0.5-cup of quinoa or dark rice. You oughtn't to avoid beans off totally on a Pegan diet. However, Hyman urges alert with them, saying that their starch substance will raise glucose. In any event, one cup of beans (or, preferably, lentils) is allowed each day. Similarly, as other distinctive clean eating consumes fewer calories, the Pegan diet downplays desserts as a rare treat.

- Dairy products: Avoid milk, yoghurt, butter and cheese, particularly if they are made from Cow is milk. Sheep or goat milk is permissible in limited quantities. It strongly discourages Cow is milk, yoghurt, and cheese. Foods derived from sheep or goat milk are, however, authorized in limited quantities. Grass-fed butter is approved occasionally, too.
- Sugar: Sparingly use it and avoid sweetened items.
- Owing to their perceived effect on blood sugar and inflammation in your body, most of these foods are prohibited.
- Grains: Gluten is strongly discouraged, but limited quantities of whole grains that are gluten-free are okay.
- Legumes: In particular, starchy legumes (including peanuts) get nixed, but lentils are tolerated.

The Pegan diet is generally plant-based, with low glycemic vegetables like broccoli and cauliflower. Grass-took care of, natural meat is permitted and subsequently is fish. Anyway, they should be considered a feature dish or fixing as opposed to the real feast. It's likewise higher to adhere to low- mercury fish like anchovies, sardines and herring. Eggs are a significant stock of protein during this eating routine, as are solid fats - coconuts, avocados, nuts (not peanuts), olive oil and Omega-three fats are completely affirmed nourishments. Nonetheless, make certain to stay eliminated from canola, sunflower oil, corn and soybean oil. Dairy, especially cow is milk and cheddar, isn't half of the eating routine. Nor is bread or elective assortments of grains; however, limited quantities of sans gluten grains are permitted. What is more, while you are permitted sugar, it ought to be eaten sparingly - anyway literally nothing prepared with added substances or additives.

Benefits of Pegan Diet
The Pegan diet may add to your well-being in various ways. The solid accentuation on leafy foods admission is maybe its best attribute. Products of the soil are some of the most healthfully different food sources. They are loaded up with fiber, nutrients, minerals, and plant intensifies known to thwart illness and lessen each oxidative pressure and irritation. The Pegan diet also stresses sound, unsaturated fats from fish, nuts, seeds, and different plants that will affect heart well-being. Besides, slims down that rely on entire nourishments and contain not many super-handed food sources are identified with improved general eating regimen quality. Albeit the Pegan diet takes into consideration more adaptability than a veggie lover or paleo diet alone, a large number of the proposed limitations pointlessly limit reliable food sources, similar to vegetables, entire grains, and dairy. Advocates of the Pegan diet normally refer to expanded irritation and raised glucose as the principal explanations behind those nourishment's expulsion. A few people do have hypersensitivities to gluten and dairy, which will advance aggravation. Essentially, certain people battle to control glucose while burning-through high-starch nourishments like grains or vegetables. Since the Pegan diet stresses supplement made natural products, vegetables, and good fats, it could encourage hinder illness, advance heart well-being, and lessen aggravation. It's basic data that a solid eating routine contains masses of soil products, and studies show most Americans are still woefully lacking in this division. A Pegan diet can fill any holes in your five-a-day target, giving a ton of-required fiber and micronutrients. The glycemic file could be a framework that estimates how singular nourishments raise blood glucose. The Pegan diet urges clients to actuate instructed concerning which food sources encourage settle this example since a yo-yo of good and bad times in glucose will have unsafe impacts. This can be positive, particularly for those with diabetes, pre-diabetes, and diverse insulin-associated conditions. The paleo diet regularly gets analysis for its negative natural effect. On the off chance that everyone ate meat at each feast, the world would confront the unfortunate aftereffects of land debasement, air contamination, and water abuse. Agnosticism mitigates this effect by empowering the acquisition of economically raised meat-and downsizing utilization ordinarily.

Let's be honest: It's hard to submit a hundred per cent to paleo or veganism.

Given its center ground between the two, the Pegan diet offers more equilibrium and adaptability. Vegetarians and paleo eaters may locate this an invite relief. In an incredible nutshell, a Pegan diet could be a high-fat, low- starch, moderate-protein method of eating that moves your body from consuming glucose (sugar) for energy to a territory of Pegan, in which your body especially utilizes solid bodies and fat as a fuel supply. Your liver makes solid bodies from fat when your body needs to make energy anyway, and no glucose is available. This cycle most normally happens during carb limitation, extremely restricted food consumption, and great exercise.

- A great many people on the planet right presently are consuming glucose as their essential wellspring of energy. This glucose is retained into your circulation system, where it triggers the arrival of insulin by your pancreas. Insulin at that point suggests the take-up of glucose by your muscles to store that glucose for use as glycogen. Insulin furthermore flags your body to store abundance glucose and fatty substances as muscle versus fat and ends any fat consuming presently happening.
- Fructose, the sugar regularly found in natural products, agave nectar, and-fairly scandalously high-fructose corn syrup (among various food sources), is handled by the liver, where it is either changed over to glucose and shipped off the circulation system (where the on top of strategy happens) or put away as fat (fatty substances) a couple of inside the liver.
- Even though an exceptionally modest quantity of fructose is changed over to fatty substances, over the long run, devouring remarkably extreme measures of fructose can prompt non-alcoholic greasy liver sickness. Inside the presence of insulin opposition, coursing glucose levels will remain too high, harming tissues, keeping the body in a very condition of fat stockpiling, and keeping the body from consuming fat that has just been put away.
- Finally, insulin obstruction will bring about a couple of diabetes, other metabolic issues, and even cardiovascular sickness. your circulation system, the release of another chemical known as glucagon is set off. Glucagon advises your liver to change over that put-away glycogen back to glucose for use as fuel. Glucagon likewise advises your body to separate put away fat into free unsaturated fats to be utilized as fuel.
- Consuming free unsaturated fats produces solid bodies, that your mind and body will use for energy.

This is the beginning of healthful Pegan. If you keep on limiting sugars, your body can keep consuming fat as its principal fuel supply. At present, something cool about sound digestion is that it removes insulin of the image. Rather than fluctuating, insulin and glucose levels remain moderately steady. This dependability checks fat stockpiling diminishes food longings and advances the breakdown of muscle to fat ratio. This straightforward fat misfortune and guideline of craving signals are among the most reasons, so a few people wind up staying with Pegan and low carb counts calories. A solid eating routine isn't the goal to anything all by itself; it ought to be applied as a feature of a sound way of life to see the most extreme outcomes. Think about the Pegan diet as the establishment of your new body. If you might want to make one thing truly exceptional on prime of it, style your way of life given that objective. Removing low-quality nourishment goes while not saying, as will dumping negative behavior patterns like smoking and drinking. Exercise, as well, can take you to statures you never thought was potential. In this way, as you investigate these delightful dishes and set out on the Pegan diet, do whatever it takes not to disregard various regions or duty. The Pegan diet advances sound, entire nourishments rich in a few of the nutrients and minerals that your body wants. Contingent upon what your present eating regimen resembles, this could prompt significant Pegan diet weight reduction. For somebody following an antiquated Western eating regimen stacked with handled nourishments, for example, the Pegan diet results might be bountiful more recognizable than for someone previously following a by and large solid eating routine. It's likewise similarly clear and easy to follow. Not at all like elective eating designs, there is no need to tally Pegan diet macros or monitor focuses, calories or carbs, which makes it a lot simpler to continue in the long haul. Additionally, the eating regimen underlines solid fixings that can improve numerous well-being past weight reduction, including heart well-being, glucose levels and illness anticipation. On the Pegan diet, sound oils, organic products, veggies, some of the best nuts, seeds and feasible wellsprings of protein are completely included. The entirety of that will be incredible increases to a balanced eating regimen.

How Pegan Diet Brings Weight Loss

One of the essential things that we tend to lose after leaving on the Pegan diet consistently is the most emphatical water weight. The body stores glucose as fat fats; however, a little glucose proposal is put away as glycogen, which comprises the main water. Glycogen should supply speedy blasting energy, the sort that we tend to might want after we are running or lifting loads. As we will cut carbs in general, the body goes to glycogen as the primary energy offer pool, which is why water weight can be lost in the underlying stages. This underlying explosion of shed pounds can be a confidence sponsor for a few, and it's a keen sign for what is to return for society who continue with the Pegan diet. On a side note, water weight is very much lost and acquired. This implies that for society who see a few outcomes on the Pegan diet at first and afterwards choose to ask off the fad for reasons unknown, the probabilities are their weight would expand duplicate once carbs turn into the day-by-day caloric backbone. For the rest of the stick with the Pegan diet, what occurs next can be the muscle versus fat is consuming component that is answerable for the shocking weight reduction results seen by many. The fundamental reason keeps on being indistinguishable. Fat fats are presently initiated as wellsprings of energy by the body's organs and cells, bringing about a characteristic condition of fat misfortune and henceforth going with weight decrease. Fat consuming isn't the solitary motivation behind why weight reduction is seen on the Pegan diet. Yearning concealment and improving satiety once suppers are why people can better fit while on the eating routine. The saying of eating less and moving extra has continually been among the long-standing principles in weight reduction. The entire arrangement is to frame a calorie shortage with the end goal that the body is needed to depend on it put away supplies of energy to shape up for the necessary consumption. On paper, that sounds simple and simple; however, for any individual who has experienced circumstances where you have needed to check your eating on a ravenous mid-region deliberately, it could be pretty much as problematic as scaling Mount Everest! With the Pegan diet, you perceive that you'll have characteristic yearning concealment, due to the change of the chemicals that administration sensations of craving and totality. Other than that, the food that we normally devour while on the eating routine additionally assists with the weight misfortune. Fats and protein are identified to be more nourishing and satisfying than sweet carbs. After we change to a high-fat eating routine though bringing down on the carbs, we will, in general, accomplish two things basically at the indistinguishable time. Moving back on carbs, particularly the sweet stuff, lessens the motivation to eat essentially because you are feeling like it, not because of your truly eager. Lifting the fat admission likewise makes the satiety impact a ton of faster and lets you are feeling full. This is half of the motivation behind why a few Pegan calorie counters say that they can continue two and a 0.5 or even two suppers consistently without feeling the smallest spot of appetite. On our Pegan feast plan, we will in the public record for a day-by-day caloric admission that goes from one,800 to two,000 calories. In general, we won't amazingly use calorie limitation to scale back weight along these lines. When you are encountering completion and fulfilment from your dinners, those little and guiltless looking tidbits that involve the time in the middle of suppers can't highlight much in your life! Think concerning it: doughnuts, chips, and cakes that are the standard go-to snacks get removed, just because you are less apparent to offer into indulgent appetite caused principally by those equivalent sweet treats! That goes a truly long methodology in cutting abundance calories that would somehow have been changed over to fat tissue. The Pegan diet licenses for suppers without the regular calorie limitation of elective weight reduction slims down to add it up. It moreover gives some assistance in making hunger concealment impacts accordingly that you don't should focus on those obnoxious cravings for food! Likewise, there is the nonappearance of carb yearnings, which can, without a doubt, crash any eating routine. This allows us to extravagant characteristic weight reduction with as almost no interruption to our day by day lives as potential. No calorie counters should be conveyed, no requirement for an inconvenient six to eight suppers every day, and decidedly no strange or entertaining activity schedules required. Having the chance to relearn what genuine craving resembles conjointly comes as another positive side project. On a carb-rich eating routine, we get occurrences of appetite because our glucose levels will, in general, hesitate fiercely as our cells become steadily insulin desensitized. Sugar conjointly expands the propensity to eat without much forethought, which will truly crash any eating routine! After we stall on carbs and increase on the fats, we would amazingly need to sit down up and pay heed once we feel any food cravings, because of those future right signals that your body needs refueling.

Summary

The Pegan diet is a ketogenic diet, that is, oriented towards the consumption of proteins and fats. The name comes from the union of the so-called paleo diet and the vegan diet. The paleo diet is inspired by the diet of our ancestors, while the vegan diet, as is well known, excludes the consumption of foods of animal origin.

In 2013 the strengths of the two diets were combined to create the Pegan diet.

Pegan diet: what you eat

The fundamental point of the Pegan diet is the exclusion of industrialized or processed foods, such as sugars or starches, favoring vegetable foods rich in healthy fats and proteins. Products of animal origin can be consumed, but care must be taken that the meat comes from outdoor and pasture farms, so that the animals are not fed with feed.

Another salient feature of the Pegan diet is the use of organic foods, fresh raw materials from organic farming, possibly grown in the most natural way possible, without chemicals, pesticides or additives.

A low carb diets

The Pegan diet is also defined as "low carb", is with few carbohydrates. This is why it is very suitable for those who need to control their blood sugar: the large consumption of vegetables - in season and possibly at kilometer 0 - together with fruit, which is also very present, helps to contain the glycemic index throughout the day.

The Pegan diet in 3 points

1. 75% of the daily food intake must be represented by fruit and vegetables.
2. 25% of the nutrition must be made up of protein, i.e., meat from extensive and environmentally friendly and vegetable farms.
3. The consumption of healthy fats, such as omega 3 contained in fish and other foods, is fundamental. Saturated fats must be present in the diet even if in not excessive percentages.

The plan for losing weight

To follow the Pegan diet for 365 days it is essential to stick to a food plan. Every day it is recommended to take the amount corresponding to at least 5 cups of vegetables, 4 of carbohydrates, 3 of proteins, 2 of fats, 1 of milk substitutes.

Here's what an example of a Pegan diet daily menu might look like:

avocado toast for breakfast; as a mid-morning snack 4-5 fresh strawberries; for lunch, a mixed salad with half a cup of legumes; as an afternoon snack a sliced cucumber or hazelnuts; for dinner a bowl of rice and cauliflower and at least 85 grams of protein.

As for alcohol, the following rule must be followed: 2 drinks per week (and with a drink we mean a glass of wine or beer). Two desserts per week are also allowed.

How to use this book

In the Pegan diet is possible to eat various foods, the important thing is to respect the daily proportions.

So, you can find in this book series of recipes divided by type of meal which, however, must be combined with each other respecting the rules of the diet. When you choose, for example, a substantial breakfast, then the subsequent meals must necessarily be lighter and substantially based on vegetable intake, such as a salad for example. The same is true if you prefer a more substantial lunch or dinner or snack.

In this book, various recipes have been proposed to help organize the diet according to the rules indicated in the introduction.

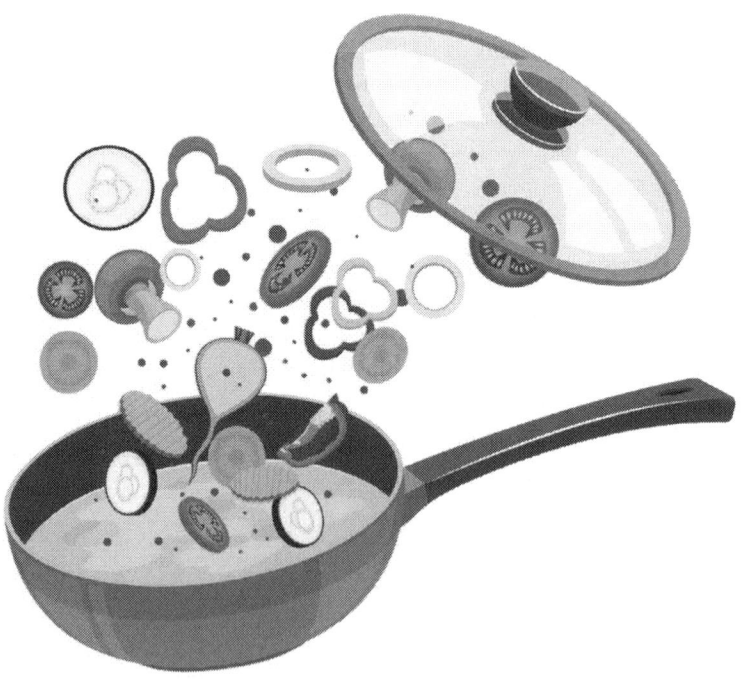

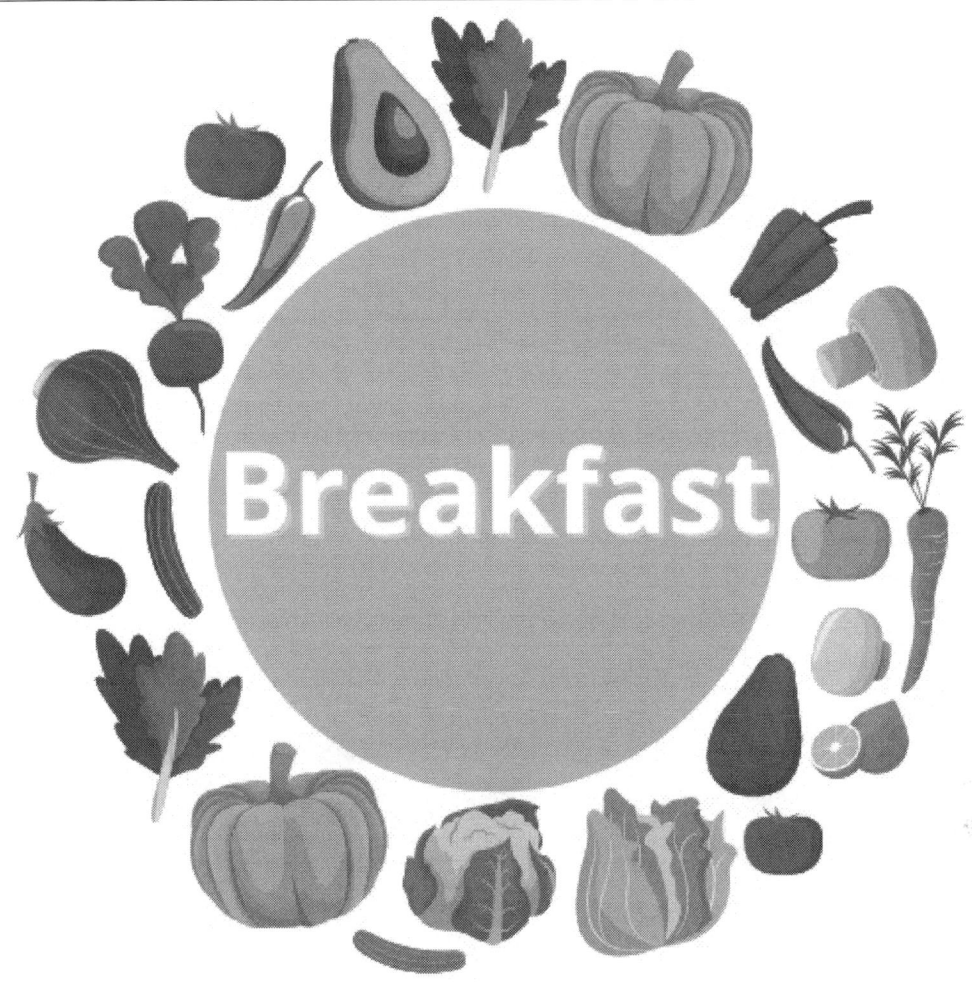

Chapter 2: Breakfast Recipes

Pegan Breakfast Pot
Instructions:

- 2 eggs, whisked
- 1 tablespoon coconut oil
- ½ tsp. smoked paprika
- 4 ounces beef, ground
- 1 yellow onion, sliced off
- 8 mushrooms, sliced
- Table salt and black pepper to the taste
- 1 avocado, pitted, peeled and sliced off
- 12 black olives, pitted and sliced

Instructions:

- Heat a dish using the coconut oil above Moderate heat, insert mushrooms, onions, pepper and table salt, prepare and shake for 5 minutes.

- Insert beef and paprika and shake fry, prepare for 10 minutes and then shift to a pot. Heat the dish up over moderate heat, insert eggs, some pepper and table salt and then scramble them. Pour beef combine to dish and shake fry.
- Insert olives and avocado, prepare and shake for 1 minute.

Eggs and Sausages with Black Pepper

Instructions:

- 12 ham slices
- 2 sausages, sliced off
- 1 yellow onion, sliced off
- 5 tbsp ghee
- 12 eggs
- Table salt and black pepper to the taste
- 1-ounce spinach, torn
- 1 red bell pepper, sliced off

Instructions:

- Heat a dish up with 1 tbsp ghee over moderate heat, insert coriander and onion, prepare and shake for 5 minutes.
- Insert bell pepper, pepper and table salt, prepare and shake for 3 minutes longer and move to a pot. Insert a piece of ham in every mug cake mold, split spinach in every and the sausage combine.
- Leave your mug cakes to cool a little before serving.

Scrambled Mushrooms Eggs

Instructions:

- 2 ham slices, sliced off
- ¼ mug red bell pepper, sliced off
- ½ mug spinach, sliced off
- 4 bell mushrooms, sliced off
- 3 eggs, whisked
- Table salt and black pepper to the taste
- 1 tablespoon coconut oil

Instructions:

- Heat a dish with half the oil over Moderate heat, insert lettuce, mushrooms, ham and bell pepper, prepare and shake for 4 minutes.
- Heat other dishes up with the remaining part of the oil over moderate heat, then insert eggs and scramble them.
- Insert ham and veggies, pepper and table salt, shake fry for 1 minute and then serve.

Delicious Spinach Frittata

Instructions:

- Table salt and black pepper to the taste
- 5 ounces mozzarella, shredded
- ½ mug parmesan, grated
- 9 ounces spinach
- 12 eggs
- 1-ounce pepperoni
- 1 tsp. garlic, chopped
- ½ mug ricotta cheese
- 4 tbsp olive oil
- A pinch of nutmeg

Instructions:

- Press liquid from spinach and put in a pot. In another pot, combine eggs with table salt, pepper, nutmeg and garlic and whisk well. Insert spinach, parmesan and ricotta and whisk well again.
- Pour this into a dish, Garnish mozzarella and pepperoni on top, introduce in the oven and bake at 375 degrees F for 45 minutes. Leave frittata to cool down for a few minutes before serving it.

Blueberries Almond Cereal

Instructions:

- 1/3 mug coconut milk
- 1 tablespoon chia seeds
- 1/3 mug water
- A handful blueberries
- 2 tbsp almonds, sliced off
- 2 tablespoon pepitas, roasted
- 1 small banana, sliced off

Instructions:

- In a pot, then combine chia seeds together with coconut milk in your food processor, combine half of those pepitas with almonds and pulse them nicely.
- Top with the remaining pepitas, banana bits and blueberries and function. Also insert the water and shake. Top with the rest of the pepitas, banana pieces and blueberries and serve.

Fruit Paleo Granola Macadamia Nuts

Ingredients:

- 2 tbsp unrefined coconut oil
- 1 mug coarsely sliced off raw almonds

- 1 mug raw macadamia nuts
- 2 tbsp unsulfured, unsweetened golden raisins
- Unsweetened almond milk or coconut milk
- 1 mug shelled raw pistachio nuts
- ½ mug unsweetened coconut chips
- ⅔ mug fresh orange juice
- 1 ½-inch piece fresh ginger, peeled and thinly sliced
- 1 tsp. green tea leaves
- ¼ mug sliced off unsulfured, unsweetened dried apricots
- 2 tbsp sliced off dried unsulfured, unsweetened stemmed dried figs

Instructions:

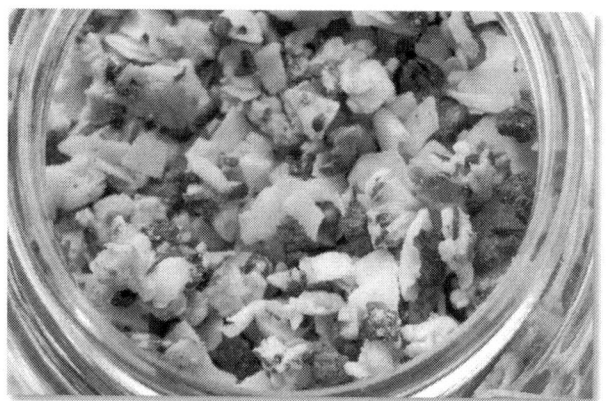

- Heat orange juice only until boiling. Insert ginger pieces. Remove from the heat; insert green tea leaves. Strain orange juice combine through a fine-mesh sieve. Remove tea leaves and ginger pieces.
- Insert coconut oil into warm lemon juice combine and shake till melted. Scatter evenly into a large skillet combine. Insert coconut chips; shake fry combine and Scatter to an even coating. Insert apricots, figs, and raisins; shake fry till well blended.
- Scatter granola on a big piece of foil or blank rimmed baking sheet; cool entirely. Serve with coconut or almond milk.

Cashews Salmon Breakfast

Instructions:

- 1 mug coconut milk
- ½ mug cashews, soaked, drained
- ¼ mug green onions, sliced off
- 4 eggs, whisked
- ½ tsp. avocado oil
- 4 ounces smoked salmon, sliced off
- 1 tsp. garlic grinding grains
- Table salt and black pepper to the taste
- 1 tablespoon lemon juice

Instructions:

- On your blender, combine cashews with coconut oil Garlic, milk grinding celery and lemon juice and combine well. Insert pepper, table salt and green onions, then combine well nicely, move to a pot and keep in the refrigerator for the time being.

- Heat a dish with the oil above moderate-low warmth, insert eggs, whisk a little and prepare till they are nearly done Introduce on your preheated broiler and prepare until eggs set. Distribute eggs plates, top with smoked salmon and function together with the green skillet on top.

Eggs Baked in Avocados with Black Pepper
Instructions:

- Table salt and black pepper to the taste
- 2 avocados, slice in halves and pitted
- 4 eggs
- 1 tablespoon chives, sliced off

Instructions:

- Scoop some flesh from the avocado halves and Organize them in a baking dish. Crack an egg in each avocado, season with table salt and pepper, introduce them in the oven at 425 degrees F and bake for 20 minutes.
- Garnish chives at the end and serve for breakfast.

Mexican Pork Breakfast
Instructions:

- Table salt and black pepper to the taste
- 8 eggs
- 1 tomato, sliced off
- ½ mug enchilada sauce
- 1-pound pork, ground
- 1-pound chorizo, sliced off
- 3 tbsp ghee
- ½ mug red onion, sliced off
- 1 avocado, pitted, peeled and sliced off

Instructions:

- In a pot, combine pork with chorizo, shake fry and Distribute onto a lined baking type. Heat a dish together with the ghee over moderate heat, insert eggs and scramble them nicely.
- Take pork combine from the oven and Scatter scrambled eggs. Garnish table salt, pepper, tomato, avocado and onion, split between plates and serve.

Special Breakfast Eggs with Tamari Sauce
Instructions:

- 2 tbsp cinnamon
- 6-star anise
- 1 tsp. black pepper

- 1 tbsp peppercorn
- 4 tea bags
- 4 tbsp table salt
- 12 eggs
- 8 mugs water
- 1 mug tamari sauce

Instructions:

- Put water into a pot, insert eggs bring them to A boil over moderate heat and prepare till they are hard boiled.
- Down them and Crack them. Insert cracked eggs, remove tea Leave eggs to cool peel and serve them.

Breakfast Pie with Mango Salsa

Instructions:

- ¾ pound beef, ground
- Table salt and black pepper to the taste
- 3 tbsp taco seasoning
- 1 tsp. baking soda
- Mango salsa for serving
- A handful cilantro, sliced off
- ½ onion, sliced off
- 1 pie crust
- ½ red bell pepper, sliced off
- 8 eggs
- 1 tsp. coconut oil

Instructions:

- Warmth up a dish with the oil over moderate warmth, insert meat, prepare until its earthy colors and blends in with table salt, pepper and taco preparing. Combine once more, move to a pot and leave aside for the time being.
- Warmth up the dish again over moderate warmth with preparing juices from the meat, insert onion and chime pepper, combine and prepare for 4 minutes. Insert eggs, preparing pop and some table salt and combine well. Insert cilantro, combine again and remove warmth. Scatter hamburger blend in pie outside layer, insert veggies blend and Scatter over meat, present in the broiler at 350 degrees F and heat for 45 minutes.
- Leave the pie to cool off a piece, slice, partition among plates and present with mango salsa on top.

Breakfast Pork Skillet

Instructions:

- 1 tablespoon coconut oil
- ½ tsp. garlic grinding grains
- ½ tsp. basil, dried
- 8 ounces mushrooms, sliced off
- Table salt and black pepper to the taste
- 1-pound pork, chopped
- 2 tbsp Dijon mustard
- 2 zucchinis, sliced off

Instructions:

- Warmth up a skillet with the oil over moderate immense warmth, insert mushrooms, combine and prepare for 4 minutes. Insert zucchinis, table salt and pepper, combine and prepare for 4 minutes more.
- Insert pork, garlic crushing grains, basil, more table salt and pepper, combine and prepare until meat is finished. Insert mustard, combine, prepare for 3 minutes more, partition into pots and serve.

Breakfast Avocado Casserole

Instructions:

- 3 mugs spinach, torn
- Table salt and black pepper to the taste
- 10 eggs
- 1-pound pork sausage, sliced off
- 1 yellow onion, sliced off
- 3 tbsp avocado oil

Instructions:

- Heat a dish with 1 tbsp oil over Insert onion, prepare and shake for 3 minutes longer. Insert spinach, prepare and shake for 1 minute. Grease a baking dish with the remainder of the oil and disperse sausage combine.
- Whisk eggs and insert them combine. Leave office to cool for a couple minutes prior to serving it for breakfast.

Amazing Breakfast Patties

Instructions:

- ½ tsp. sage, dried
- ¼ tsp. ginger, dried
- 3 tablespoon cold water
- 1-pound pork meat, chopped

- Table salt and black pepper to the taste
- ¼ tsp. thyme, dried
- 1 tablespoon coconut oil

Instructions:

- In a different pot, combine Insert this to beef and shake really well. Shape your patties and set them onto a working surface.
- Heat a dish using the coconut oil on moderate immense heat, then insert patties, fry them for 5 minutes, then flip and prepare them for 3 minutes longer. Serve them warm.

Breakfast Dish

Instructions:

- ¼ mug coconut milk
- 6 asparagus stalks, sliced off
- 1 tablespoon dill, sliced off
- 1-pound sausage, sliced off
- 1 leek, sliced off
- 8 eggs, whisked
- Table salt and black pepper to the taste
- ¼ tsp. garlic grinding grains
- 1 tablespoon coconut oil, melted

Instructions:

- Heat a dish over moderate heat, insert sausage Bits and brown them for a couple of minutes. Insert asparagus and leek, prepare and shake for a couple of minutes.
- Pour it into a baking dish that you've greased using the coconut oil. Insert veggies and sausage on top and liquefy all. Drink warm.

Lean and Green Cauliflower Breakfast

Instructions:

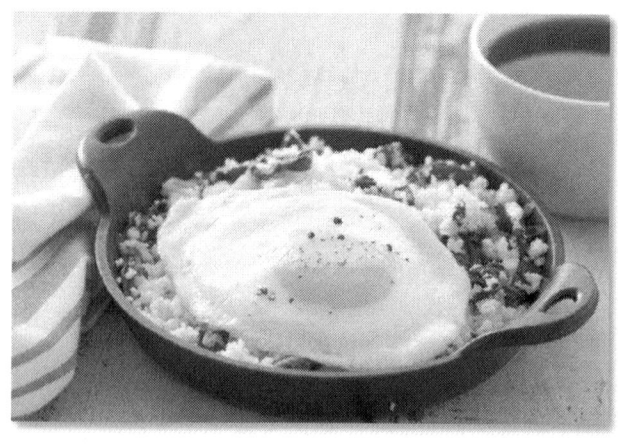

- ½ tsp. garlic grinding grains
- Table salt and black pepper to the taste
- 1 cauliflower head, florets separated
- 4 eggs, whisked
- 1-pound chorizo, sliced off
- 12 ounces canned green chilies, sliced off
- 1 yellow onion, sliced off
- 2 tbsp green onions, sliced off

Instructions:

- Heat a dish over moderate heat, insert chorizo and onion, brown and shake for a couple of minutes.
- On your food processor blend cauliflower with some pepper and table salt and combine. Shift this into a pot, then insert eggs, table salt, garlic and pepper and scatter everything. Insert chorizo combine too, whisk again and again move all to a greased baking dish.

Onion Breakfast Hash

Ingredients:

- Table salt and black pepper to the taste
- 1 yellow onion, sliced off
- 2 mugs corned beef, sliced off
- 1 tablespoon coconut oil
- 2 garlic cloves, chopped
- ½ mug beef stock
- 1-pound radishes, slice in quarters

Instructions:

- Warm up a dish with the oil over moderate immense heat, insert onion, shake and prepare for 4 minutes. Insert radishes, shake and prepare for 5 minutes. Insert garlic, shake and prepare for 1 minute more.
- Insert stock, beef, table salt and pepper, shake, prepare for 5 minutes, remove heat and serve.

Breakfast Beef Meat Shake Fry

Instructions:

- 2 bell peppers, sliced off
- 1 tsp. chili grinding grains
- 1 tablespoon coconut oil
- 2 eggs
- Table salt and black pepper to the taste
- ½ pounds beef meat, chopped
- 2 teaspoons red chili flakes
- 1 tablespoon tamari sauce
- 6 bunches book choy, trimmed and sliced off
- 1 tsp. ginger, grated
- Table salt to the taste

Instructions:

- Heat a pot with 1 tbsp coconut oil Insert pepper, table salt, tamari sauce, chili flakes and chili grinding nuts, shake fry, prepare for 4 minutes longer and take heat off.
- Heat another dish up with 1 tbsp oil over moderate heat, insert publication choy, prepare and shake for 3 minutes. Insert ginger and table salt, shake fry, prepare for two minutes longer

and take heat off. Warm up the next dish with 1 tbsp oil over moderate heat, crack eggs and fry them. Split steak and bell peppers blend into two pots.

Medifast Breakfast Porridge
Instructions:

- 1 tsp. stevia
- ¾ mug coconut cream
- A pinch of cardamom, ground
- 1 tsp. cinnamon grinding grains
- A pinch of nutmeg
- ½ mug almonds, ground
- A pinch of cloves, ground

Instructions:

- Warm up a dish over moderate heat, insert coconut cream and Warm up for a few minutes. Insert stevia and almonds and shake well for 5 minutes.
- Insert cloves, cardamom, nutmeg and cinnamon and shake well. Shift to a pot and serve warm.

Almonds Breakfast Pot
Instructions:

- 1 tsp. pistachios, sliced off
- 1 tsp. pine nuts, raw
- 1 tsp. sunflower seeds, raw
- 1 tsp. pecans, sliced off
- 1 mug coconut milk
- 1 tsp. walnuts, sliced off
- 1 tsp. raw honey
- 1 tsp. pepitas, raw
- 1 tsp. almonds, sliced off
- 2 teaspoons raspberries

Instructions:

- Heat a dish over moderate heat, insert coconut Cream and heat to get a couple of minutes. Insert stevia and almonds and shake fry for 5 minutes.
- Shift into a pot and pour warm.

Breakfast Coconut Muffins
Ingredients:

- Table salt and black pepper to the taste
- ¼ mug kale, sliced off

- 8 prosciutto slices
- ½ mug almond milk
- 6 eggs
- 1 tablespoon coconut oil
- ¼ mug chives, sliced off

Instructions:

- In a pot, combine eggs with table salt, pepper, milk, chives and kale and shake well. Grease a muffin tray with melted coconut oil, line with prosciutto slices, pour eggs combine, introduce in the oven and bake at 350 degrees F for 30 minutes.
- Shift muffins to a platter and serve for breakfast
- for 15 minutes. Serve these tasty breads.

Chicken Breakfast Muffins

Ingredients:

- ½ tsp. garlic grinding grains
- 3 tbsp warm sauce combined with 3 tbsp melted coconut oil
- 6 eggs
- ¾ pound chicken breast, boneless
- Table salt and black pepper to the taste
- 2 tbsp green onions, sliced off

Instructions:

- Shift chicken breast into a pot, then shred with a fork and combine with half the sauce and melted coconut oil. Fling to coat and then leave aside for now.
- In a pot, combine eggs with table salt, pepper, green onions and the remainder of the warm sauce blended with oil and whisk nicely. Drink your muffins sexy.

Avocado Black Pepper Muffins

Ingredients:

- 1 mug coconut milk
- 2 mugs avocado, pitted, peeled and sliced off
- Table salt and black pepper to the taste
- ½ tsp. baking soda
- 4 eggs
- 6 bacon slices, sliced off
- 1 yellow onion, sliced off
- ½ mug coconut flour

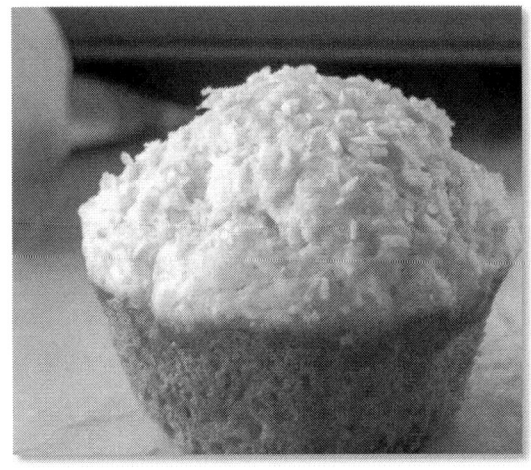

Instructions:

- Heat a dish over moderate heat, insert onion and bacon, brown and shake for a couple of minutes. Insert milk, pepper, table salt, baking soda and coconut milk and shake fry everything.
- Insert bacon combine and shake. Grease a muffin tray using the coconut oil, then split avocado and eggs blend into the menu, present from the oven at 350 degrees F and bake for 20 minutes. Distribute muffins between dishes and serve them.

Bacon and Lemon Muffins

Ingredients:

- 3 mugs almond flour
- 1 tsp. baking soda
- 4 eggs
- 1 mug bacon, finely sliced off
- Table salt and black pepper to the taste
- ½ mug ghee, melted
- 2 teaspoons lemon thyme

Instructions:

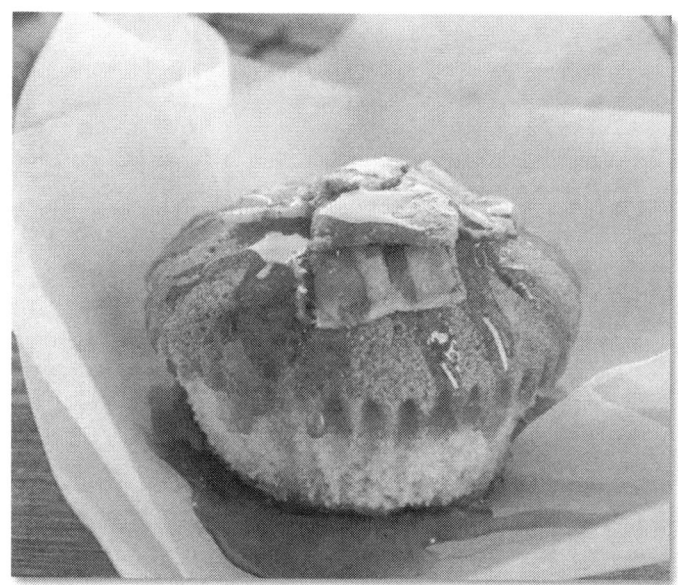

- In a pot, combine flour with baking soda and eggs and shake well. Insert ghee, lemon thyme, bacon, table salt and pepper and whisk well. Distribute this into a lined muffin dish, introduce in the oven at 350 degrees F and bake for 20 minutes.
- Leave muffins to cool down a bit, distribute between plates and serve them.

Almond and Oregano Muffins

Ingredients:

- ½ tsp. oregano, dried
- 1 mug almond flour
- ¼ tsp. baking soda
- Table salt and black pepper to the taste
- ½ mug coconut milk
- 2 tbsp olive oil
- 1 egg
- 2 tbsp parmesan cheese
- 1 mug cheddar cheese, grated

Instructions:

- In a pot, combine flour with oregano, table salt, pepper, parmesan and baking soda and shake. In another pot, combine coconut milk with egg and olive oil and shake well. Combine the 2 combinators and whisk well. Insert cheddar cheese, shake, pour this a lined muffin tray, introduce in the oven at 350 degrees F for 25 minutes.
- Leave your muffins to cool down for a few minutes, distribute them between plates and serve.

Amazing Turkey Breakfast

Ingredients:

- 2 bacon sliced
- 2 turkey breast slices, already prepared
- 2 avocado slices
- Table salt and black pepper
- 2 tbsp coconut oil
- 2 eggs, whisked

Instructions:

- Heat a dish over moderate heat, insert bacon pieces and brown them for a couple of minutes. Meanwhile, heating a different dish with the petroleum Over moderate heat, insert eggs, pepper and table salt and scramble them.
- Split turkey Breast pieces on two plates. Distribute scrambled eggs. Split bacon pieces and avocado pieces also and function.

Paprika Burrito

Ingredients:

- ¼ pound beef meat, ground
- 1 tsp. sweet paprika
- 1 tsp. onion grinding grains
- 1 small red onion, julienned
- 1 tsp. coconut oil
- 1 tsp. garlic grinding grains
- 1 tsp. cumin, ground
- 1 tsp. cilantro, sliced off
- Table salt and black pepper to the taste
- 3 eggs

Instructions:

- Heat a dish over moderate heat, insert beef and brown for a couple of minutes. Insert pepper, table salt, cumin, garlic and garlic grinding grains and paprika, shake fry for 4 minutes longer and take heat off. Put in a pot, combine eggs with pepper and table salt and whisk well.

- Heat a dish with the oil over moderate heat, insert egg, then Scatter evenly and prepare for 6 minutes. Shift your egg burrito into a plate, then split beef combine, insert celery and onion, roll up and serve.

Fueling Granola
Instructions:

- A splash of lemon juice
- 2 tbsp pecans, sliced off
- 2 tbsp chocolate, sliced off
- 7 strawberries, sliced off

Instructions:

- In a pot, combine chocolate with strawberries, pecans and lemon juice. Shake and serve cold.

Shrimp and Bacon Breakfast
Instructions:

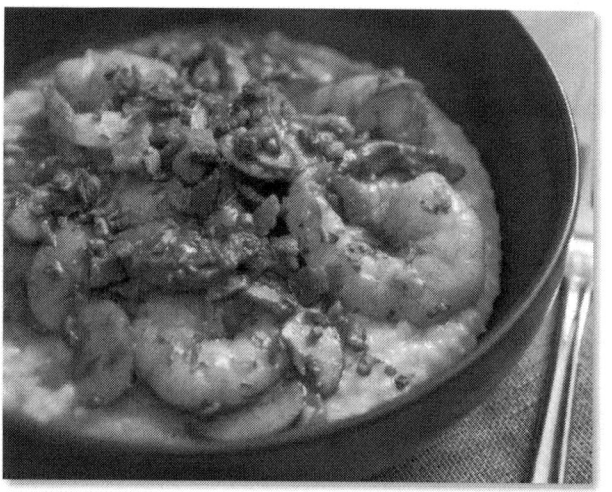

- 4 ounces smoked salmon, sliced off
- 4 ounces shrimp, deveined
- 1 mug mushrooms, sliced
- 4 bacon slices, sliced off
- Table salt and black pepper to the taste
- ½ mug coconut cream

Instructions:

- Heat a dish over moderate heat, insert bacon, Prepare and shake for 5 minutes. Insert mushrooms, prepare and shake for 5 minutes longer.
- Insert salmon, prepare and shake for 3 minutes. Insert fish and prepare for two minutes. Insert pepper, table salt and coconut cream, shake fry 1 minute, eliminate heat and split between dishes.

Brussels Bacons Sprouts
Ingredients:

- 2 shallots, chopped
- 2 garlic cloves, chopped
- 12 ounces Brussels sprouts, thinly sliced
- 2 ounces bacon, sliced off
- 3 eggs
- Table salt and black pepper to the taste

- 1 tablespoon ghee, melted
- 1 and ½ tbsp apple cider vinegar

Instructions:

- Heat a dish over moderate heat, insert bacon, Shake, prepare till it is crispy, move to a plate and leave aside for now. Heat the dish up over moderate heat, then insert shallots and garlic, then prepare and shake for 30 minutes. Insert Brussels sprouts, pepper, table salt and apple cider vinegar, prepare and shake for 5 minutes.
- Pour bacon to dish, then prepare and shake for 5 minutes longer. Insert ghee, shake and make a hole at the middle. Crack eggs to the dish, then prepare until they are done and serve instantly.

Breakfast Cereal Nibs
Ingredients:

- 1 tablespoon vanilla extract
- 1 tablespoon psyllium grinding grains
- 2 tbsp coconut oil
- 4 tbsp hemp hearts
- ½ mug chia seeds
- 1 mug water
- 1 tablespoon swerve
- 2 tbsp cocoa nibs

Instructions:

- In a pot, then combine chia seeds with water, shake fry Insert hemp hearts, vanilla extract, psyllium grinding grains, oil and shake well with your own combiner. Insert cocoa nibs and shake fry till you get a dough. Distribute dough into two pieces, form into cylinder form, put onto a lined baking sheet, flatten well, wrap up with a parchment paper, then introduce from the oven at 285 degrees F and bake for 20 minutes.
- Take cylinders from the oven, leave aside to cool and slice into little pieces. Serve at the morning with some almond milk.

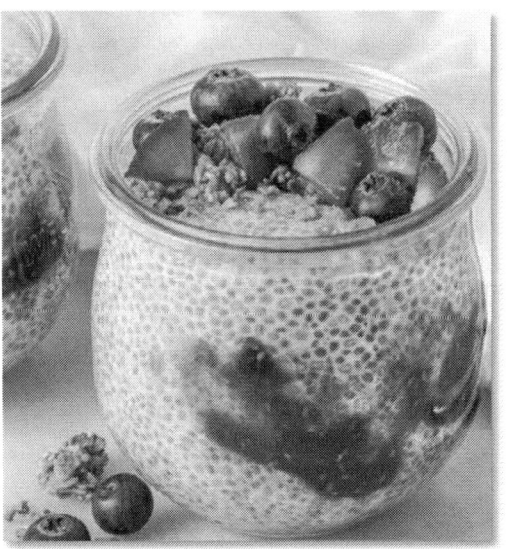

Chia Pudding
Ingredients:

- 1 tablespoon swerve
- 1 tablespoon vanilla extract
- 2 tbsp cocoa nibs
- 2 tbsp coffee
- 2 mugs water
- 1/3 mug chia seeds
- 1/3 mug coconut cream

Instructions:

- Heat a little pot with water above Moderate heat, bring to a boil, insert java, simmer for 15 minutes, remove heat and strain into a pot. Insert vanilla extract, coconut lotion, swerve, cocoa nibs and chia seeds, shake well, keep in the refrigerator for half an hour, split into two breakfast pots and function.

Tasty Hemp Porridge
Ingredients:

- ½ mug hemp hearts
- ½ tsp. cinnamon, ground
- 1 tablespoon stevia
- 1 tablespoon chia seeds
- 1 mug almond milk
- 2 tbsp flax seeds
- ¾ tsp. vanilla extract
- ¼ mug almond flour
- 1 tablespoon hemp hearts for serving

Instructions:

- In a pot, combine almond milk using 1/2 mug hemp Prepare for two minutes, then remove heat, insert vanilla milk, shake well and pour into a pot. Top with 1 tbsp hemp hearts and function.

Steak and Eggs
Ingredients:

- 3 eggs
- 1 tablespoon ghee
- 4 ounces sirloin
- 1 small avocado, pitted, peeled and sliced
- Table salt and black pepper to the taste

Instructions:

- Heat a dish together with the ghee over moderate Immense warmth, crack eggs into the dish and then prepare them as you desire. Season with pepper and table salt, eliminate heat and shift to a plate. Heat another dish over moderate immense heat, then include sirloin, prepare for 4 minutes, then remove heat, leave aside to cool and slice into thin strips.
- Season with pepper and table salt into the flavor and put beside the eggs. Insert avocado slices on both sides and function.

Egg Porridge

Ingredients:

- 1/3 mug heavy cream
- 2 tbsp ghee, melted
- 2 eggs
- 1 tablespoon stevia
- A pinch of cinnamon, ground

Instructions:

- In a pot, combine eggs with stevia and heavy cream and whisk well. Warm up a dish with the ghee over moderate immense heat, insert egg combine and prepare until they are done.
- Shift to 2 pots, Garnish cinnamon on top and serve.

Almond Dish cakes

Ingredients:

- 1/3 mug coconut, shredded
- ½ tsp. baking grinding grains
- 1 mug almond milk
- ¼ mug coconut oil
- 1 tsp. almond extract
- 6 eggs
- A pinch of table salt
- ½ mug coconut flour
- ¼ mug stevia
- ¼ mug almonds, toasted
- 2 ounces cocoa chocolate
- Preparing spray

Instructions:

- Put in a pot, combine coconut milk with stevia, insert almonds and chocolate and whisk well. Heat a dish with preparing spray over moderate heat, then insert tablespoon batter, Scatter to a circle, then prepare till it is golden, flip, prepare until it is done and move to a dish.
- Repeat with the remaining portion of the batter and then serve your dish cakes straight away.

Amazing Pumpkin Dish cakes

Ingredients:

- 1 tsp. baking grinding grains
- 1 mug coconut cream
- 3 eggs
- 5 drops stevia
- 1 tablespoon swerve

- 1 tablespoon chai masala
- 1 tsp. vanilla extract
- 1-ounce egg white protein
- 2 ounces hazelnut flour
- 2 ounces flax seeds, ground
- ½ mug pumpkin puree
- 1 tsp. coconut oil

Instructions:

- In a pot, then combine flax seeds using hazelnut in a different pot, combine coconut cream with vanilla extract, pumpkin puree, eggs, stevia and shake well.
- Combine both combinators and shake well. Heat a dish with the oil over moderate immense heat, then pour 1/6 of this batter, then Scatter into a circle, wrap up, reduce heat to low, prepare 3 minutes on each side and shift to a plate. Repeat with the remaining portion of the batter and then serve your sausage sandwiches straight away.

Breakfast French Toast

Ingredients:

- 1 mug whey protein
- 1 tsp. cinnamon, ground
- ½ mug ghee, melted
- ½ mug almond milk
- ½ mug swerve
- 12 egg whites
- 1 tsp. vanilla
- ½ mug coconut milk
- 2 eggs

Instructions:

- In a pot, then combine 12 egg whites together with your Combiner for a couple of minutes. Insert protein and shake lightly. Insert cream cheese and shake. Pour this into two greased bread dishes, then introduce from the oven at 325 degrees F and bake for 45 minutes. Leave breads to cool and slit them into 18 pieces. In a pot combine 2 eggs vanilla, cinnamon and coconut milk and whisk well.
- Dip bread slices in this combine. Heat a dish with a few coconut oils over moderate heat, insert bread pieces, prepare till they are golden on each side and then split between plates. Heat a dish together with all the ghee over immense heat, then insert vanilla milk and Warm up nicely. Insert swerve, shake and take heat off. Leave aside to cool a little and drizzle over French toasts.

Baked Granola

Ingredients:

- ½ mug coconut, flaked
- ¼ mug flax meal
- ½ mug almond milk
- 1 tsp. vanilla
- 1 tsp. cinnamon, ground
- A pinch of table salt
- ¼ mug sunflower seeds
- ¼ mug pepitas
- ½ mug almonds, sliced off
- 1 mug pecans, sliced off
- ½ mug walnuts, chopped
- ½ mug stevia
- ¼ mug ghee, melted
- 1 tsp. honey
- ½ tsp. nutmeg
- ¼ mug water

Instructions:

- In a pot, combine almonds with pecans, grease a baking sheet with parchment paper, then disperse granola blend and press nicely. Wrap up with another piece of parchment paper, then introduce from the oven at 250 degrees F and bake for 1 hour.
- Take granola from the oven, leave aside to cool, break into pieces and serve.

Amazing Breakfast Smoothie

Ingredients:

- 2 mugs spinach leaves
- 1 tsp. green grinding grains
- 1 tsp. whey protein
- 2 brazil nuts
- 1 mug coconut milk
- 10 almonds
- 1 tablespoon psyllium seeds
- 1 tablespoon potato starch

Instructions:

- In your blender, combine spinach with brazil nuts, coconut milk and almonds and blend well. Insert green grinding grains, whey protein, potato starch and psyllium seeds and blend well again. Pour into a tall glass and consume for breakfast.

Breakfast Lean and Green Smoothie

Ingredients:

- 1 tablespoon ginger, grated
- 1 tablespoon swerve
- 1 mug cucumber, sliced
- 1 mug lettuce leaves
- 4 mugs water
- 2 tbsp parsley leaves
- ½ avocado, pitted and peeled
- ½ mug kiwi, peeled and sliced
- 1/3 mug pineapple, sliced off

Instructions:

- In your blender, combine water with lettuce leaves, pineapple, parsley, cucumber, ginger, kiwi, avocado and swerve and blend very well. Pour into glasses and serve for a breakfast.

Delightful Chicken Quiche

Ingredients:

- Table salt and black pepper to the taste
- 2 zucchinis, grated
- ½ mug heavy cream
- 1 tsp. fennel seeds
- 7 eggs
- 2 mugs almond flour
- 2 tbsp coconut oil
- 1 tsp. oregano, dried
- 1-pound chicken meat, ground

Instructions:

- In your food processor, combine almond milk Using a pinch of table salt. Insert 1 egg and coconut oil and combine well. Put dough in a greased pie dish and press nicely on the ground.
- Heat a dish over moderate heat, insert chicken meat, brown for a few minutes, then remove heat and leave aside. In a pot, combine 6 eggs with pepper, table salt, peppermint, lotion and fennel seeds and scatter well.
- Insert chicken meat and shake fry. Pour it into pie crust, disperse, introduce from the oven at 350 degrees F and bake for 40 minutes. Leave the dish to cool a little before slicing and serving it for breakfast.

Chicken Omelet

Ingredients:

- 1 tomato, sliced off
- 2 bacon slices, prepared and crumbled
- 2 eggs
- 1 small avocado, pitted, peeled and sliced off
- 1-ounce rotisserie chicken, shredded
- 1 tsp. mustard
- 1 tablespoon homemade mayonnaise
- Table salt and black pepper to the taste

Instructions:

- In a pot, combine eggs with some table salt and Pepper and whisk lightly. Heat a dish over moderate heat, spray some preparing oil, then insert eggs and prepare your omelet for 5 minutes. Insert chicken, avocado, celery, tomato, mayo and mustard on one half of the omelet.

Delicious Green Smoothie Pot

Ingredients:

- ½ mug almond milk
- 1 tsp. protein grinding grains
- 4 raspberries
- 2 ice cubes
- 1 tablespoon coconut oil
- 2 tbsp heavy cream
- 1 mug spinach
- 1 tablespoon coconut, shredded
- 4 walnuts
- 1 tsp. chia seeds

Instructions:

- In your blender, combine milk with spinach, cream, ice, protein grinding grains and coconut oil, blend well and shift to a pot. Top your pot with raspberries, coconut, walnuts and chia seeds and serve.

Tuna Salad Breakfast

Ingredients:

- Table salt and black pepper to the taste
- A pinch of chili flakes
- 2 tbsp sour cream
- 12 ounces tuna in olive oil

- 4 leeks, finely sliced off
- 1 tablespoon capers
- 8 tbsp homemade mayonnaise

Instructions:

- In a salad pot, combine tuna with capers, table salt, pepper, leeks, chili flakes, sour cream and mayo. Shake well and serve with some crispy bread.

Breakfast Salad in A Jar
Ingredients:

- 4 ounces rotisserie chicken, roughly sliced off
- 4 tbsp extra virgin olive oil
- ½ scallion, sliced off
- 1-ounce favorite greens
- 1-ounce red bell pepper, sliced off
- 1-ounce cherry tomatoes, halved
- 1-ounce cucumber, sliced off
- Table salt and black pepper to the taste

Instructions:

- In a pot, combine greens with bell pepper, tomatoes, scallion, cucumber, table salt, pepper and olive oil and fling to coat well. Shift this to a jar, top with chicken pieces and serve for breakfast.

Salmon Patties and Zucchini Ribbons
Ingredients:

- 2 tbsp thinly sliced scallions
- 1 tsp. Mexican Seasoning
- Black pepper
- 10 ounces prepared salmon
- 2 egg whites
- ½ mug almond flour
- ⅓ mug shredded sweet potato
- 4 tbsp olive oil
- Tomatillo-Mango Salsa (see recipe, below)
- 2 tbsp snipped fresh cilantro
- 2 tbsp Chipotle Paleo Mayo
- 1 tablespoon fresh lime juice
- 1 ripe avocado, peeled, seeded, and sliced

Instructions:

- For salmon patties, at a large pot using a Fork to flake grilled salmon into little pieces. Combine lightly to blend. Distribute combine into eight parts; shape each portion into a patty. (Cakes could be cooled 1 day before serving.) In a large nonstick skillet heat 2 tablespoon olive oil on moderate-immense heat. Insert half of those cakes into the skillet; prepare about 8 minutes or till golden brown, turning the cakes halfway through preparing.
- Shift the cakes into a different parchment-lined baking sheet and keep warm from the oven. Fry the rest of the cakes at the remaining 2 tablespoons oil as directed. To serve, Organize Zucchini Ribbons at a nest on all four serving dishes.
- Top each with two salmon sandwiches, a poached egg, a number of those Tomatillo-Mango Salsa, and avocado slices.

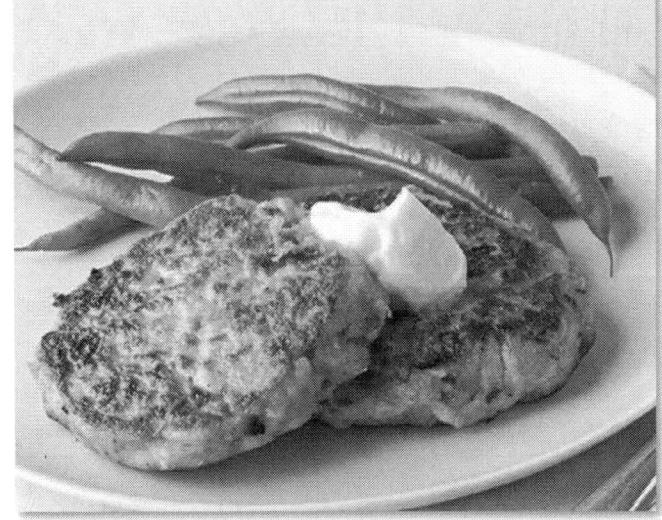

Poached Eggs

Ingredients:

- 2 tbsp white vinegar
- 4 large eggs, each cracked into small, handled mug
- Table salt and pepper

Instructions:

- Fill 8-to 10-inch nonstick skillet virtually to rim with water, then insert 1 tsp. table salt and vinegar, and then bring to boil over large heat. Lower lip of every mug into water once; hint eggs into boiling water, wrap up, and remove from heat.
- Poach eggs 4 minutes for moderate-firm yolks, 4 minutes to get firmer yolks, or 3 minutes to get looser yolks.
- With slotted spoon, carefully lift and drain every egg. Season with pepper and table salt to taste and serve instantly.

Foolproof Hard-Prepared Eggs

Ingredients:

- 4 large eggs

Instructions:

- Put eggs in moderate sauce dish, wrap up with 1-inch water, and bring to boil over immense heat. Remove dish from heat, wrap up, and let sit 10 minutes. Meanwhile, fill moderate pot with 4 mugs water and 1 tray of ice cubes. Shift eggs to ice water bath with slotted spoon; let sit for 5 minutes. Peel eggs.

Butter Scrambled Eggs

Ingredients:

- Table salt
- 1 tsp. pepper
- 8 large eggs plus 2 large yolks
- 1 mug half-and-half
- 1 tablespoon unable salted butter, cooled

Instructions:

- And one tsp. pepper with fork until completely blended and combine is pure yellow; don't overbeat. Melt butter 10-inch nonstick skillet over moderate-immense heat until foaming just subsides (butter shouldn't brown), swirling to coat dish.
- Insert egg combine and, with heatproof rubber spatula, always and securely scrape along sides and bottom of skillet until eggs start to clump and spatula leaves path on bottom of 1 1 to 2 2 minutes. Reduce heat to low and gently but always fold eggs till clumped and only slightly moist, 30 to 60 minutes.
- Instantly move eggs to heated plates and season with table salt to taste. Drink instantly.

Eggs with Asparagus and Parmesan

Ingredients:

- 1 tsp. pepper
- 1 tsp. vegetable oil
- 1 tablespoon unable salted butter
- 12 large eggs
- 6 tbsp half-and-half
- 3/ tsp. table salt
- 3 ounces thinly sliced prosciutto, slice into 1 -inch pieces
- 1-ounce Parmesan cheese, grated (1 mug)
- 8 ounces asparagus, trimmed, halved lengthwise, and slice on bias into 1 -inch lengths

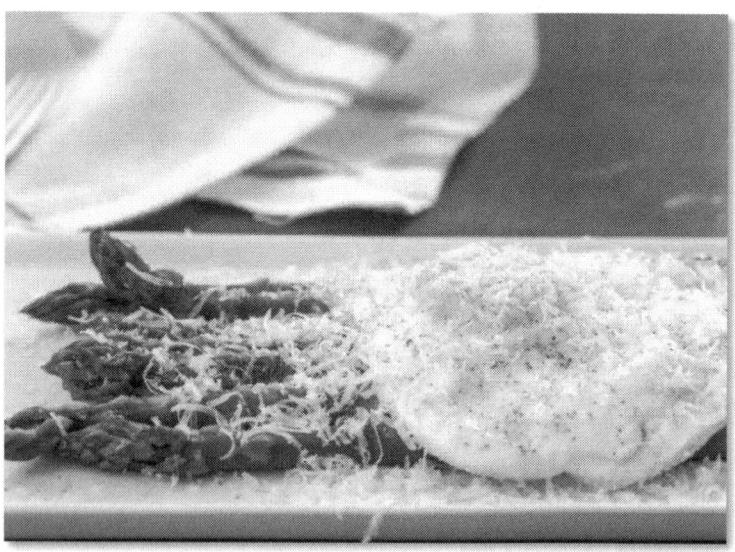

Instructions:

- With fork in moderate pot until completely blended. Heat oil at 12-inch Skillet over moderate heat until shimmering. minutes. Scatter asparagus in single layer on moderate plate; Put aside. Wipe out Insert butter into now-empty skillet and melt over moderate Pour egg combine. Together with heatproof rubber spatula, shake eggs slowly pushing them from side to side, scratching along Bottom and sides of skillet, and folding and lifting eggs since they form curds (don't over-scramble eggs or curds are going to probably be too modest).

- Prepare until big curds Shape but eggs are still quite moist, 2-3 minutes. Off heat, gently fold Prosciutto, Parmesan, and asparagus until evenly dispersed; if eggs are still Underdone, return skillet to moderate heat for no more than 30 minutes. Distribute eggs among individual plates and serve instantly.

Eggs with Sausage and Cheddar

Ingredients:

- 12 large eggs
- 1 tsp. vegetable oil
- 8 ounces sweet Italian sausage, casings removed, sausage crumbled into 1 -inch pieces
- 1 red bell pepper, stemmed, seeded, and slice into 1 -inch pieces
- 3 scallions, white and green parts separated, both sliced thin on bias
- 6 tbsp half-and-half
- 3/tsp. table salt
- 1 tsp. pepper
- 1 tablespoon unable salted butter
- 1 1 ounce's sharp cheddar cheese, shredded (1 mug)

Instructions:

- Beat eggs, half-and-half, table salt, and pepper with fork in moderate pot until thoroughly combined. Heat oil in 12-inch nonstick skillet over moderate heat until shimmering. Insert sausage and prepare, breaking into 1 -inch pieces until beginning to brown, about 2 minutes. Insert bell pepper and scallion whites; continue to prepare, shake ring occasionally, until sausage is prepared through and pepper is beginning to brown, about 3 minutes. Scatters combine in single layer on moderate plate; set aside.
- Wipe out skillet with paper towels. Insert butter to now-empty skillet and melt over moderate heat, swirling to coat dish. Pour in egg combine.
- With heatproof rubber spatula, shake eggs constantly, slowly pushing them from side to side, scraping along bottom and sides of skillet, and lifting and folding eggs as they form curds (do not over scramble or curds formed will be too small). Prepare until large curds form but eggs are still very moist, 2 to 3 minutes.
- Off heat, gently fold in sausage combine and cheddar until evenly distributed; if eggs are still underdone, return skillet to moderate heat for no longer than 30 seconds. Distribute eggs among individual plates, Garnish with scallion greens, and serve instantly.

Fried Eggs

Ingredients:

- 1 tablespoon unable salted butter, cooled
- 4 large eggs
- Table salt and pepper

Instructions:

- Heat 10-inch nonstick skillet over low heat for 5 minutes. Meanwhile, crack open 2 eggs into mug or small pot: crack remaining 2 eggs into second mug or small pot. Insert butter to skillet, let melt, and swirl to coat dish. Working quickly, pour 2 eggs into skillet on one side and remaining 2 eggs on opposite side.
- Season eggs with table salt and pepper to taste, wrap up, and prepare about 2 1 minutes for runny yolks, 3 minutes for soft but set yolks, or 3 1 minutes for firmly set yolks. Slide eggs onto plate; serve.

Classic Filled Omelet

Ingredients:

- 1 tablespoon unable salted butter, plus melted butter for brushing omelet
- 3 tbsp finely shredded Gruyere cheese
- 3 large eggs
- Table salt and pepper

Instructions:

- Beat eggs and table salt and pepper to taste with fork in small pot until thoroughly combined. Melt butter in 10-inch nonstick skillet over moderate-immense heat. Insert eggs and prepare until edges begin to set, 2 to 3 seconds. Using heatproof rubber spatula, shake in circular motion until slightly thickened, about 10 seconds. Use spatula to pull prepared edges in toward center, then tilt dish to one side so that unprepared eggs run to edge of dish. Repeat until omelet is just set but still moist on surface, 20 to 25 seconds. Garnish Gruyere and filling down center of omelet.
- Remove skillet from burner. Using rubber spatula, fold lower third (portion nearest you) of omelet over filling; press gently with spatula to secure seams, maintaining fold. Run spatula between outer edge of omelet and dish to loosen. Jerk dish sharply toward you a few times to slide omelet up far side of dish. Jerk dish again so that unfolded edge folds over itself or use spatula to fold edge over. Invert omelet onto plate. Tidy edges with spatula, brush with melted butter, and serve.

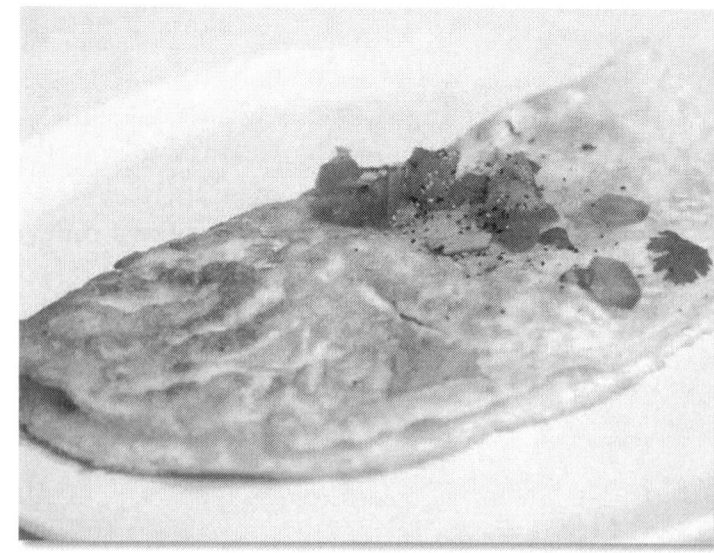

Asparagus Omelet

Ingredients:

- Table salt and pepper
- 1 shallot, halved and sliced thin
- 1 tsp. lemon juice
- 2 tbsp unable salted butter
- 8 ounces asparagus, trimmed and slice on bias into 1 -inch pieces
- 5 large eggs
- 1 1 ounces Gruyere cheese, shredded fine (1 mug)

Instructions:

- Melt 1 tablespoon butter in 10-inch nonstick skillet over moderate immense heat. Insert asparagus, pinch table salt, and pepper to taste and prepare, shake ring occasionally, for 2 minutes. Insert shallot and prepare, shake ring occasionally, until asparagus is lightly browned and tender, 2 to 4 minutes longer. Insert lemon juice and fling to coat; shift to pot. Meanwhile, beat eggs and table salt and pepper to taste with fork in small pot until combined. Wipe skillet clean with paper towel.
- Melt remaining 1 tablespoon butter in now-empty skillet over moderate-low heat. Insert eggs and prepare, without shake ring, until eggs begin to set, 45 to 60 seconds. Using heatproof rubber spatula and working around edge of entire dish, lift edge of prepared egg, then tilt dish to one side so that unprepared eggs run underneath; gently scrape unprepared eggs toward rim of skillet, until top is just slightly wet, 1 1 to 2 minutes. Let dish sit without moving for 30 seconds. Off heat, Garnish asparagus combine in even layer over omelet, then Garnish cheese evenly over asparagus.
- Wrap up and let sit until eggs no longer appear wet, 4 to 5 minutes. Return skillet to moderate heat for 30 seconds. Using rubber spatula, loosen edges of omelet from skillet. Slide omelet halfway out of dish onto serving plate. Tilt dish so top of omelet folds over itself. Slice omelet in half and serve instantly.

Delightful French Omelets

Ingredients:

- 1 tsp. table salt
- Pepper
- 2 tbsp unable salted butter, slice into 2 pieces
- 1 tsp. vegetable oil
- 6 large eggs, cooled
- 2 tbsp shredded Gruyere cheese
- 4 teaspoons chopped fresh chives

Instructions:

- Slice 1 tablespoon butter in half. Slice remaining 1 tablespoon butter into small pieces, shift to small pot, and Put in freezer while preparing eggs and skillet, at least 10 minutes.

Meanwhile, heat oil in 8- inch nonstick skillet over low heat for 10 minutes. Crack 2 eggs into moderate pot and separate third egg; reserve egg white for another use and insert egg yolk to pot.

- Insert table salt and pinch pepper. Break egg yolks with fork, then beat eggs at moderate pace, about 80 strokes, until yolks and whites are well combined. Shake in half of frozen butter cubes. When skillet is fully heated, use paper towels to wipe out oil, leaving thin film on bottom and sides of skillet. Insert 1 tablespoon of reserved butter to skillet and heat until melted. Swirl butter to coat skillet, insert egg combine, and expand heat to moderate-immense. Use 2 chopsticks or wooden skewers to scramble eggs, using quick circular motion to move around skillet, scraping prepared egg from side of skillet as you go, until eggs are almost prepared but still slightly runny, 45 to 90 seconds.

- Turn off heat (remove skillet from heat if using electric burner) and smooth eggs into even layer using heatproof rubber spatula. Garnish omelet with 1 tablespoon Gruyere and 2 teaspoons chives.

- Wrap up skillet with tight-fitting lid and let sit for 1 minute for runnier omelet or 2 minutes for firmer omelet. Heat skillet over low heat for 20 seconds, unwrap up, and, using rubber spatula, loosen edges of omelet from skillet. Put folded square of paper towel onto warmed plate and slide omelet out of skillet onto paper towel so that omelet lies flat on plate and hangs about 1 inch off paper towel. Roll omelet into neat cylinder and set aside. Return skillet to low heat and heat for 2 minutes before repeating instructions for second omelet starting with step 2. Serve.

Garlic Mayonnaise Dip

Ingredients:

- 1 garlic clove, chopped
- ¾ mug vegetable oil
- 1 tablespoon water
- 2 large egg yolks
- 2 teaspoons Dijon mustard
- 2 teaspoons lemon juice
- 1 mug extra-virgin olive oil
- 1 tsp. table salt
- 1 tsp. pepper

Instructions:

- Process egg yolks, mustard, lemon juice, and garlic in food processor until combined, about 10 seconds. With processor running, slowly drizzle in vegetable oil, about 1 minute. Shifts combine to moderate pot and whisk in water.

- Whisking constantly, slowly drizzle in olive oil, about 30 seconds. Whisk in table salt and pepper. (Mayonnaise can be refrigerated for up to 4 days.)

Trout with Sweet Potatoes

Ingredients:

- 3 tbsp refined coconut oil
- 1½ pounds white or yellow sweet potatoes, peeled
- Refined coconut oil for frying
- sliced off fresh parsley
- 4 6-ounce fresh or frozen skinless trout fillets, ¼ to ½ inch thick
- 1½ teaspoons Smoky Seasoning
- ¼ to ½ tsp. black pepper (optional)
- Sliced scallions

Instructions:

- Preheat oven to 400°F. Thaw fish, if frozen. Rinse fish; pat dry with paper towels. Garnish fillets with Smoky Seasoning and, if desired, pepper. In an extra-large oven going skillet heat 2 tbsp of the oil over moderate-immense heat. Put fillets in skillet and bake, unwrap upped, for 6 to 8 minutes or until fish begins to flake when tested with a fork.
- Remove from oven. Meanwhile, using a julienne peeler or mandolin fitted with the julienne slicer, slice sweet potatoes lengthwise into long thin strips. Wrap potato strips in a double thickness of paper towels and absorb any excess water. In a large stockpot with at least 8-inch-tall sides, heat 2 to 3 inches of refined coconut oil to 365°F.
- Carefully insert potatoes, about one-fourth at a time, to the warm oil. (Oil will rise in the pot.) Fry about 1 to 3 minutes per batch or until just starting to brown, shake ring once or twice. Quickly remove potatoes using a long-slotted spoon and drain on paper towels. (Potatoes can overprepare quickly, so check early and often.) Be sure to heat oil back up to 365°F before inserting each batch of potatoes. Garnish trout with parsley and scallions; serve with sweet potato shoestrings.

Apple-Flax Jacks

Ingredients:

- ¼ mug finely sliced off walnuts or pecans
- 2 teaspoons finely shredded orange peel
- ½ mug almond butter
- 2 teaspoons finely shredded orange peel
- ¼ tsp. ground cardamom or cinnamon
- 1 tsp. pure vanilla extract
- 4 large eggs, lightly beaten
- 2 large, unpeeled apples, cored and finely shredded
- ½ mug flax meal
- 1 tsp. ground cardamom or cinnamon
- 3 tbsp unrefined coconut oil

Instructions:

- In a large pot combine eggs, shredded apples, flax meal, nuts, orange peel, vanilla, and 1 tsp. cardamom. Shake until well combined. Let batter stand for 5 to 10 minutes to thicken. On a griddle or skillet melt 1 tablespoon of the coconut oil over moderate heat. For each Apple-Flax Jack, drop about ⅓ mug batter the griddle, Scattering slightly.
- Prepare over moderate heat for 3 to 4 minutes on each side or until jacks are golden brown. Meanwhile, in a small microwave-safe pot heat almond butter on low until Scatter able. Serve on top of Apple-Flax Jacks and Garnish with orange peel and cardamom.

Amazing Breakfast Cocoa Nibs

Ingredients:

- 1 mug water
- 1 mug cherries, frozen
- ¼ mug cocoa grinding grains
- 10 ounces canned coconut milk
- 1 mug favorite greens
- ¼ mug cocoa nibs
- 1 small avocado, pitted and peeled
- ¼ tsp. turmeric

Instructions:

- In your blender, combine coconut milk with avocado, cocoa grinding grains, cherries and turmeric and blend well. Insert water, greens and cocoa nibs, blend for 2 minutes more, pour into glasses and serve.

Peaches with Toasted Coconut-Almond Crunch

Ingredients:

- ½ tsp. ground cinnamon
- 1 mug unsweetened coconut flakes
- 1 mug coarsely sliced off raw almonds
- ¼ mug unable salted raw sunflower seeds
- 1 tablespoon fresh lemon juice
- 6 ripe peaches
- ½ mug unsweetened, unsulfured dried peaches, finely sliced off
- ¾ mug fresh orange juice
- ¼ mug unrefined coconut oil
- 1 vanilla bean, split and seeds scraped
- 1 mug raspberries, blueberries, blackberries, and/or coarsely sliced off strawberries

Instructions:

- In a huge sauce dish bring 8 mugs water to bubbling. Utilizing a sharp blade, cut a shallow X on the lower part of each peach. Drench peaches, two all at once, in bubbling water for 30 to 60 seconds or until skins start to part. Utilizing an opened spoon, move peaches to an enormous pot of ice water. At the point when sufficiently cool to deal with, utilize a blade or your fingers to strip off skins; eliminate skins.

- Cut peaches into wedges, eliminating the pits; put in a safe spot. Preheat broiler to 250°F. Line a huge preparing sheet with material paper. In a food processor or blender consolidate 1 cup of the peach wedges, the dried peaches, ¼ cup of the squeezed orange, the coconut oil, and cinnamon. Wrap up and cycle or mix until smooth; put in a safe spot. In an enormous pot join the coconut pieces, almonds, and sunflower seeds.
- Addition pureed peach join. Throw to cover. Move nut consolidate to the readied heating sheet, Scattering equally.
- Prepare for 60 to 75 minutes or until dry and fresh, shake ring at times. (Be mindful so as not to consume; join will fresh up additional as it cools.) Meanwhile, Put the leftover peach wedges into a moderate substantial sauce dish. Shake in the excess ½ mug squeezed orange, the lemon squeeze, and split vanilla bean (with seeds). Bring to bubbling over moderate warmth, shake ring once in a while. Lessen warmth to low; stew, open up increased, for 10 to 15 minutes or until thickened, shake ring every so often.
- Eliminate vanilla bean unit. Shake in berries. Get ready for 3 to 4 minutes or just until berries are warmed through.

Poached Eggs

Instructions:

- Table salt and black pepper to the taste
- 1 red bell pepper, sliced off
- 3 tomatoes, sliced off
- 1 tsp. paprika
- 1 tsp. cumin
- 3 garlic cloves, chopped
- 1 tablespoon ghee
- 1 white onion, sliced off
- 1 Serrano pepper, sliced off
- ¼ tsp. chili grinding grains
- 1 tablespoon cilantro, sliced off
- 6 eggs

Instructions:

- Warm up a dish with the ghee over moderate heat, insert onion, shake and prepare for 10 minutes. Insert Serrano pepper and garlic, shake and prepare for 1 minute. Insert red bell pepper, shake and prepare for 10 minutes.
- Insert tomatoes, table salt, pepper, chili grinding grains, cumin and paprika, shake and prepare for 10 minutes. Crack eggs into the dish, season them with table salt and pepper, wrap up dish and prepare for 6 minutes more. Garnish cilantro at the end and serve.

Strawberry-Mango Power Smoothies

Ingredients:

- 1¼ mugs unsweetened coconut milk or almond milk
- ¼ mug unsweetened pomegranate juice
- ¼ mug unable salted almond butter
- 1 moderate red beet, peeled and quartered (about 4 ounces)
- 2½ mugs hulled fresh strawberries
- 1½ mugs frozen unsweetened mango chunks
- 2 teaspoons egg white grinding grains

Instructions:

- In a moderate sauce dish prepare beet, Wrap upped, in a small amount of boiling water for 30 to 40 minutes or until very tender. Drain beet; run cold water over beet to cool quickly. Drain well. In a blender combine beet, strawberries, mango chunks, coconut milk, pomegranate juice, and almond butter.
- Wrap up and blend until smooth, stopping to scrape sides of blender as needed. Insert egg white grinding grains. Wrap up and blend just until combined. Shift frozen mango pieces to an airtight container; freeze for up to 3 months.

Date Shakes

Ingredients:

- 2 tbsp almond butter
- 1 tablespoon egg white grinding grains
- 1 tablespoon unsweetened cocoa grinding grains (optional)
- ½ tsp. fresh lemon juice
- ⅓ mug sliced off, pitted Medjool dates
- 1 mug unsweetened almond or coconut milk (with vanilla if desired)
- 1 ripe banana, frozen and sliced
- ⅛ to ¼ tsp. ground nutmeg

Instructions:

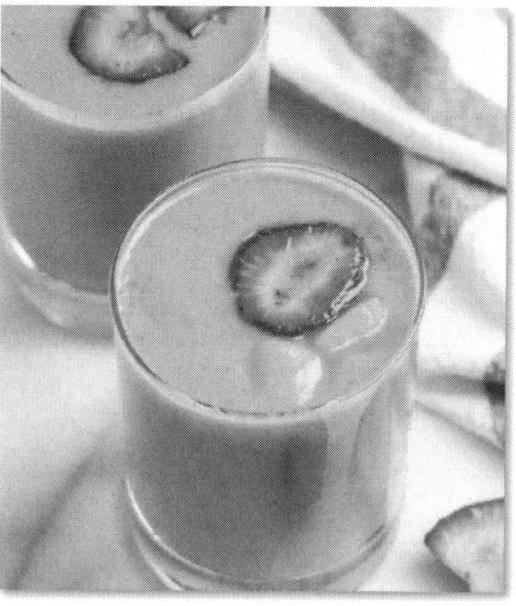

- In a small pot combine date and ½ mug water. Microwave on immense for 30 seconds or until dates are softened; drain off water.
- In a blender combine the dates, almond milk, banana slices, almond butter, egg white grinding grains, cocoa grinding grains (if using), lemon juice, and nutmeg. Wrap up and blend until smooth.

Apple chai Smoothie

Ingredients:

- 1 cup unsweetened rice milk
- 1 chai tea bag
- 1 apple, peeled, cored, and chopped
- 2 cups ice

Instructions:

- In a medium saucepan, heat the rice milk over low heat for about 5 minutes or until steaming.
- Remove the milk from the heat and add the tea bag to steep.
- Let the milk cool in the refrigerator with the tea bag for about 30 minutes
- and then remove tea bag, squeezing gently to release all the flavor.
- Place the milk, apple, and ice in a blender and blend until smooth.
- Pour into 2 glasses and serve.

Blueberry Pineapple Smoothie

Ingredients:

- 1 cup frozen blueberries
- ½ cup pineapple chunks
- ½ cup English cucumber
- ½ apple
- ½ cup water

Instructions:

- Put the blueberries, pineapple, cucumber, apple, and water in a blender and
- blend until thick and smooth.
- Pour into 2 glasses and serve.

Watermelon Raspberry Smoothie

Ingredients:

- ½ cup boiled, cooled, and shredded red cabbage
- 1 cup diced watermelon
- ½ cup fresh raspberries
- 1 cup ice

Instructions:

- Put the cabbage in a blender and pulse for 2 minutes or until it is finely chopped.
- Add the watermelon and raspberries and pulse for about 1 minute or until very well combined.
- Add the ice and blend until the smoothie is very thick and smooth.
- Pour into 2 glasses and serve.

Festive Berry Parfait

Ingredients:

- 1 cup vanilla rice milk, at room temperature
- ½ cup plain cream cheese, at room temperature
- 1 tablespoon granulated sugar
- ½ teaspoon ground cinnamon
- 1 cup crumbled Meringue Cookies (here)
- 2 cups fresh blueberries
- 1 cup sliced fresh strawberries

Instructions:

- In a small bowl, whisk together the milk, cream cheese, sugar, and cinnamon until smooth.
- Into 4 (6-ounce) glasses, spoon ¼ cup of crumbled cookie in the bottom of each.
- Spoon ¼ cup of the cream cheese mixture on top of the cookies.
- Top the cream cheese with ¼ cup of the berries.
- Repeat in each cup with the cookies, cream cheese mixture, and berries.
- Chill in the refrigerator for 1 hour and serve.

Mixed Grain Hot Cereal

Ingredients:

- 2¼ cups water
- 1¼ cups vanilla rice milk
- 6 tablespoons uncooked bulgur
- 2 tablespoons uncooked whole buckwheat
- 1 cup peeled, sliced apple
- 6 tablespoons plain uncooked couscous
- ½ teaspoon ground cinnamon

Instructions:

- In a medium saucepan over medium-high heat, heat the water and milk.
- Bring to a boil, and add the bulgur, buckwheat, and apple.
- Reduce the heat to low and simmer, stirring occasionally, for 20 to 25 minutes or until the bulgur is tender.
- Remove the saucepan from the heat and stir in the couscous and cinnamon.
- Let the saucepan stand, covered, for 10 minutes, then fluff the cereal with a fork before serving.

Corn Pudding

Ingredients:

- Unsalted butter, for greasing the baking dish
- 2 tablespoons all-purpose flour
- ½ teaspoon Ener-G baking soda substitute
- 3 eggs
- ¾ cup unsweetened rice milk, at room temperature
- 3 tablespoons unsalted butter, melted
- 2 tablespoons light sour cream

- 2 tablespoons granulated sugar
- 2 cups frozen corn kernels, thawed

Instructions:

- Preheat the oven to 350°F.
- Lightly grease an 8-by-8-inch baking dish with butter; set aside.
- In a small bowl, stir together the flour and baking soda substitute; set aside.
- In a medium bowl, whisk together the eggs, rice milk, butter, sour cream, and sugar.
- Stir the flour mixture into the egg mixture until smooth.
- Add the corn to the batter and stir until very well mixed.
- Spoon the batter into the baking dish and bake for about 40 minutes or until
- the pudding is set.
- Let the pudding cool for about 15 minutes and serve warm.

Rhubarb Bread Pudding

Ingredients:

- Unsalted butter, for greasing the baking dish
- 1½ cups unsweetened rice milk
- 3 eggs
- ½ cup granulated sugar
- 1 tablespoon cornstarch
- 1 vanilla bean, split
- 10 thick pieces white bread, cut into 1-inch chunks
- 2 cups chopped fresh rhubarb

Instructions:

- Preheat the oven to 350°F.
- Lightly grease an 8-by-8-inch baking dish with butter; set aside.
- In a large bowl, whisk together the rice milk, eggs, sugar, and cornstarch.
- Scrape the vanilla seeds into the milk mixture and whisk to blend.
- Add the bread to the egg mixture and stir to completely coat the bread.
- Add the chopped rhubarb and stir to combine.
- Let the bread and egg mixture soak for 30 minutes.
- Spoon the mixture into the prepared baking dish, cover with aluminum foil, and bake for 40 minutes.
- Uncover the bread pudding and bake for an additional 10 minutes or until the pudding is golden brown and set.
- Serve warm.

Cinnamon Nutmeg Blueberry Muffins

Ingredients:

- 2 cups unsweetened rice milk
- 1 tablespoon apple cider vinegar
- 3½ cups all-purpose flour
- 1 cup granulated sugar
- 1 tablespoon Ener-G baking soda substitute
- 1 teaspoon ground cinnamon

- ½ teaspoon ground nutmeg
- Pinch ground ginger
- ½ cup canola oil
- 2 tablespoons pure vanilla extract
- 2½ cups fresh blueberries

Instructions:

- Preheat the oven to 375°F.
- Line the cups of a muffin pan with paper liners; set aside.
- In a small bowl, stir together the rice milk and vinegar; set aside for 10 minutes.
- In a large bowl, stir together the flour, sugar, baking soda substitute,
- cinnamon, nutmeg, and ginger until well mixed. Add the oil and vanilla to the milk mixture and stir to blend.
- Add the milk mixture to the dry ingredients and stir until just combined.
- Fold in the blueberries. Spoon the muffin batter evenly into the cups.
- Bake the muffins for 25 to 30 minutes or until golden and a toothpick
- inserted in the center of a muffin comes out clean.
- Allow the muffins to cool for 15 minutes before serving.

Egg in the Hole

Ingredients:

- 2 (½-inch-thick) slices Italian bread
- ¼ cup unsalted butter
- 2 eggs
- 2 tablespoons chopped fresh chives
- Pinch cayenne pepper
- Freshly ground black pepper

Instructions:

- Using a cookie cutter or a small glass, cut a 2-inch round from the center of each piece of bread.
- In a large nonstick skillet over medium-high heat, melt the butter.
- Place the bread in the skillet, toast it for 1 minute, and then flip the bread over.
- Crack the eggs into the holes the center of the bread and cook for about 2 minutes or until the eggs are set and the bread is golden brown.
- Top with chopped chives, cayenne pepper, and black pepper.
- Cook the bread for another 2 minutes.
- Transfer an egg-in-the-hole to each plate to serve.

Summer Vegetable Omelet

Ingredients:

- 4 egg whites
- 1 egg
- 2 tablespoons chopped fresh parsley
- 2 tablespoons water
- Olive oil spray, for greasing the skillet
- ½ cup chopped and boiled red bell pepper

- ¼ cup chopped scallion, both green and white parts
- Freshly ground black pepper

Instructions:

- In a small bowl, whisk together the egg whites, egg, parsley, and water until well blended; set aside.
- Generously spray a large nonstick skillet with olive oil spray and place it over medium-high heat.
- Sauté the peppers and scallion for about 3 minutes or until softened.
- Pour the egg mixture into the skillet over the vegetables and cook, swirling
- the skillet, for about 2 minutes or until the edges of the egg start to set.
- Lift up the set edges and tilt the pan so that the uncooked egg can flow underneath the cooked egg.
- Continue lifting and cooking the egg for about 4 minutes or until the omelet is set.
- Loosen the omelet with a spatula and fold it in half. Cut the folded omelet into 3 portions and transfer the omelets to serving plates.
- Season with black pepper and serve.

Egg and Veggie Muffins

Ingredients:

- Cooking spray, for greasing the muffin pans
- 4 eggs
- 2 tablespoons unsweetened rice milk
- ½ sweet onion, finely chopped
- ½ red bell pepper, finely chopped
- 1 tablespoon chopped fresh parsley
- Pinch red pepper flakes
- Pinch freshly ground black pepper

Instructions:

- Preheat the oven to 350°F.
- Spray 4 muffin pans with cooking spray; set aside.
- In a large bowl, whisk together the eggs, milk, onion, red pepper, parsley,
- red pepper flakes, and black pepper until well combined.
- Pour the egg mixture into the prepared muffin pans.
- Bake 18 to 20 minutes or until the muffins are puffed and golden.
- Serve warm or cold.

Curried Egg Pita Pockets

Ingredients:

- 3 eggs, beaten
- 1 scallion, both green and white parts, finely chopped
- ½ red bell pepper, finely chopped
- 2 teaspoons unsalted butter
- 1 teaspoon curry powder
- ½ teaspoon ground ginger
- 2 tablespoons light sour cream

- 2 (4-inch) plain pita bread pockets, halved
- ½ cup julienned English cucumber
- 1 cup roughly chopped watercress

Instructions:

- In a small bowl, whisk together the eggs, scallion, and red pepper until well blended.
- In a large nonstick skillet over medium heat, melt the butter.
- Pour the egg mixture into the skillet and cook for about 3 minutes or until
- the eggs are just set, swirling the skillet but not stirring. Remove the eggs from the heat; set aside.
- In a small bowl, stir together the curry powder, ginger, and sour cream until well blended.
- Evenly divide the curry sauce among the 4 halves of the pita bread, spreading it out on one inside edge.
- Divide the cucumber and watercress evenly between the halves.
- Spoon the eggs into the halves, dividing the mixture evenly, to serve.

Dilly Scrambled Eggs

Ingredients:

- 2 large eggs
- 1/8 teaspoon black pepper
- 1 teaspoon dried dill weed
- 1 tablespoon crumbled goat cheese

Instructions:

- Beat the eggs in a bowl; pour them into a nonstick skillet over medium heat.
- Add black pepper and dill weed to eggs.
- Cook until eggs are scrambled.
- Top with crumbled goat cheese before serving.

Great Way to Start your Day Bagel

Ingredients:

- 1 bagel, 2-ounce size
- 2 tablespoons cream cheese
- 2 tomato slices, 1/4" thick
- 2 red onion slices
- 1 teaspoon low-sodium lemon pepper seasoning

Instructions:

- Slice bagel and toast until golden brown.
- Spread cream cheese over each bagel half. Place onion slice and tomato slice on top and sprinkle with lemon pepper.

Quick and easy Apple Oatmeal Custard

Ingredients:

- 1/3 cup quick-cooking oatmeal
- 1 large egg
- 1/2 cup almond milk
- 1/4 teaspoon cinnamon
- 1/2 medium apple

Instructions:

- Core and finely chop apple half.
- Combine oats, egg and almond milk in a large mug. Stir well with a fork. Add cinnamon and apple. Stir again until fully mixed.
- Cook in microwave on high for 2 minutes. Fluff with a fork. Cook an additional 30 to 60 seconds if needed.
- Stir in a little more milk or water if thinner cereal is desired.

Chapter 3: Lunch Recipes

Lean and Green Lunch Tacos
Ingredients:

- 2 teaspoons sriracha sauce
- ¼ mug tomatoes, sliced off
- Preparing spray
- 2 mugs cheddar cheese, grated
- 1 small avocado, pitted, peeled and sliced off
- 1 mug favorite taco meat, prepared
- Table salt and black pepper to the taste

Instructions:

- Splash some planning oil on lined preparing dish. Dissipate cheddar on the preparing sheet, present in the broiler at 400 degrees F and heat for 15 minutes. Dissipate taco meat over cheddar and prepare for 10 minutes more.
- In the interim, in a pot, join avocado with tomatoes, sriracha sauce, table salt and pepper and shake. Disperse this over taco and cheddar layers, leave tacos to chill off a piece, cut utilizing a pizza slicer and serve for lunch.

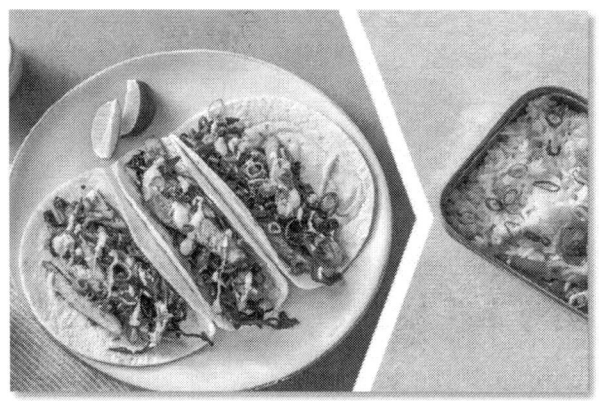

Marinara Stuffed Peppers

Ingredients:

- ½ tsp. herbs de Provence
- 1-pound sweet sausage, sliced off
- 3 tbsp yellow onions, sliced off
- Some marinara sauce
- 4 big banana peppers, tops slice off, seeds removed and slice into halves
- lengthwise
- 1 tablespoon ghee
- Table salt and black pepper to the taste
- A drizzle of olive oil

Instructions:

- Season banana peppers with table salt and pepper, drizzle the oil, rub well and bake in the oven at 350 degrees F for 20 minutes. Meanwhile, Warm up a dish over moderate heat, insert sausage pieces, shake and prepare for 5 minutes. Insert onion, herbs de Provence, table salt, pepper and ghee, shake well and prepare for 5 minutes.
- Take peppers out of the oven, fill them with the sausage combine, put them in an oven-proof dish, drizzle marinara sauce over them, introduce in the oven again and bake for 10 minutes more. Serve warm.

Lunch Burgers

Ingredients:

- 1 tablespoon garlic, chopped
- 1 tablespoon Italian seasoning
- 2 tbsp mayonnaise
- 1 tablespoon ghee
- 2 tbsp olive oil
- 1-pound brisket, ground
- 1-pound beef, ground
- Table salt and black pepper to the taste

- 8 butter slices
- 1 yellow onion, sliced off
- 1 tablespoon water

Instructions:

- In a pot, combine brisket with beef, table salt, pepper, Italian seasoning, garlic and mayo and shake well. Shape 8 patties and make a pocket in each. Stuff each burger with a butter slice and seal.
- Warm up a dish with the olive oil over moderate heat, insert onions, shake and prepare for 2 minutes. Insert the water, shake and gather them in the corner of the dish. Put burgers in the dish with the onions and prepare them over moderate-low heat for 10 minutes. Flip them, insert the ghee and prepare them for 10 minutes more. Distribute burgers on buns and serve them with caramelized onions on top.

Zucchini Dish
Ingredients:

- 1 tsp. red pepper flakes
- 1 tablespoon garlic, chopped
- 1 tablespoon red bell pepper, sliced off
- Table salt and black pepper to the taste
- 1 tablespoon basil, sliced off
- 1 tablespoon olive oil
- 3 tbsp ghee
- 2 mugs zucchini, slice with a spiralizer
- ¼ mug asiago cheese, shaved
- ¼ mug parmesan, grated

Instructions:

- Warm up a dish with the oil and ghee over moderate heat, insert garlic, bell pepper and pepper flakes, shake and prepare for 1 minute. Insert zucchini noodles, shake and prepare for 2 minutes more. Insert basil, parmesan, table salt and pepper, shake and prepare for a few seconds more. Remove heat, shift to a pot and serve for lunch with asiago cheese on top.

Bacon and Zucchini Salda
Ingrediente:

- 1/3 mug thick cheese dressing
- ½ mug bacon, prepared and crumbled
- 1 mug baby spinach
- 4 mugs zucchini noodles
- 1/3 mug bleu cheese, crumbled
- Black pepper to the taste

Instructions:

- In a salad pot, combine spinach with zucchini noodles, bacon and bleu cheese and fling. Insert cheese dressing and black pepper to the taste, fling well to coat, distribute into 2 pots and serve.

Mayonnaise Chicken Salad

Ingredients:

- 5 ounces chicken breast, roasted and sliced off
- 2 tbsp parsley, sliced off
- ½ tbsp dill relish
- Table salt and black pepper to the taste
- 1/3 mug mayonnaise
- 1 green onion, sliced off
- 1 celery rib, sliced off
- 1 egg, hard-boiled, peeled and sliced off
- A pinch of granulated garlic
- 1 tsp. mustard

Instructions:

- In your food processor, combine parsley with onion and celery and pulse well. Shift these to a pot and leave aside for now.
- Put chicken meat in your food processor, blend well and insert to the pot with the veggies. Insert egg pieces, table salt and pepper and shake. Also insert mustard, mayo, dill relish and granulated garlic, fling to coat and serve right away.

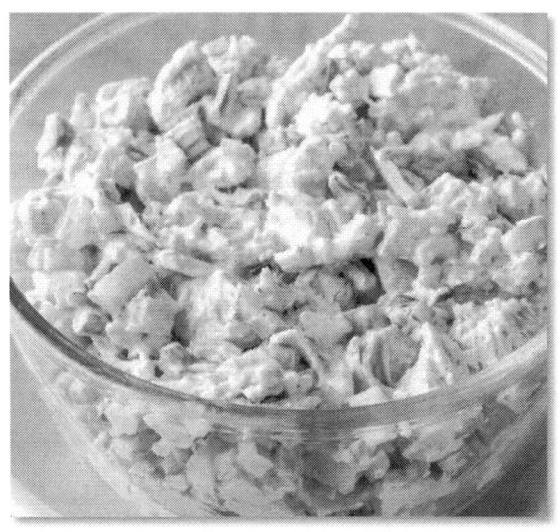

Green and Lean Steak Salad

Ingredients:

- 6 ounces sweet onion, sliced off
- 1 lettuce head, sliced off
- 2 garlic cloves, chopped
- 1 yellow bell pepper, sliced
- 1 orange bell pepper, sliced
- 1 tsp. Italian seasoning
- 4 ounces mushrooms, sliced
- 1 and ½ pound steak, thinly sliced

- 3 tbsp avocado oil
- Table salt and black pepper to the taste
- ¼ mug balsamic vinegar
- 1 avocado, pitted, peeled and sliced
- 3 ounces sun-dried tomatoes, sliced off
- 1 tsp. red pepper flakes
- 1 tsp. onion grinding grains

Instructions:

- In a pot, consolidate steak pieces with some table salt, pepper and balsamic vinegar, hurl to cover and leave aside until further notice. Warm up a dish with the avocado oil over moderate-low warmth, embed mushrooms, garlic, table salt, pepper and onion, shake and get ready for 20 minutes. In a pot, join lettuce leaves with orange and yellow chime pepper, sun dried tomatoes and avocado and shake red. Season steak pieces with onion granulating grains, pepper drops and Italian flavoring.
- Put steak pieces in a searing dish, present in preheated grill and get ready for 5 minutes. Appropriate steak pieces on plates, embed lettuce and avocado serving of mixed greens as an afterthought and top everything with onion and mushroom join.

Fennel and Chicken Lunch Salad

Ingredients:

- 1 and ½ mug fennel, sliced off
- 2 tbsp lemon juice
- ¼ mug mayonnaise
- 2 tbsp fennel fronds, sliced off
- 3 chicken breasts, boneless, skinless, prepared and sliced off
- 2 tbsp walnut oil
- ¼ mug walnuts, toasted and sliced off
- Table salt and black pepper to the taste
- A pinch of cayenne pepper

Instructions:

- In a pot, combine fennel with chicken and walnuts and shake. In another pot, combine mayo with table salt, pepper, fennel fronds, walnut oil, lemon juice, cayenne and garlic and shake well. Pour this over chicken and fennel combine, fling to coat well and keep in the fridge until you serve.

Pegan Caesar Salad

Ingredients:

- 3 tbsp creamy Caesar dressing
- 1 mug bacon, prepared and crumbled
- 1 avocado, pitted, peeled and sliced

- Table salt and black pepper to the taste
- 1 chicken breast, grilled and shredded

Instructions:

- In a salad pot, combine avocado with bacon and chicken breast and shake. Insert Caesar dressing, table salt and pepper, fling to coat, distribute into 2 pots and serve.

Easy Stuffed Avocado
Ingredients:

- 1 tablespoon mayonnaise
- 1 tablespoon lemon juice
- Table salt and black pepper to the taste
- 1 avocado
- 4 ounces canned sardines, drained
- 1 spring onion, sliced off
- ¼ tsp. turmeric grinding grains

Instructions:

- Slice avocado in halves, scoop flesh and put in a pot. Mash with a fork and combine with sardines. Mash again with your fork and combine with onion, lemon juice, turmeric grinding grains, table salt, pepper and mayo. Shake everything and Distribute into avocado halves. Serve for lunch right away.

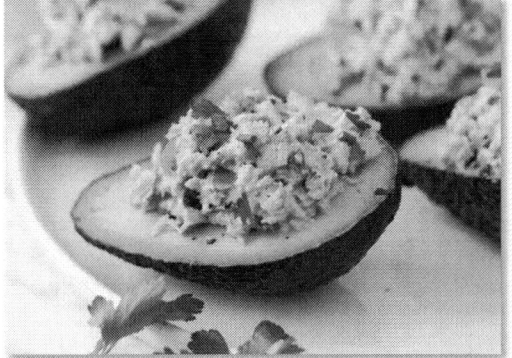

Garlic Chicken Salad
Ingredients:

- 6 bacon slices, prepared and crumbled
- ¼ mug mayonnaise
- 1 avocado, pitted, peeled and cubed
- 1-pound chicken meat, prepared and cubed
- Table salt and black pepper to the taste
- 10 cherry tomatoes, halved
- 2 tbsp garlic pesto

Instructions:

- In a salad pot, combine chicken with bacon, avocado, tomatoes, table salt and pepper and shake. Insert mayo and garlic pesto, fling well to coat and serve.

Lunch Crab Cakes

Ingredients:

- ¼ mug cilantro, sliced off
- 1 tsp. jalapeno pepper, chopped
- 1 tsp. lemon juice
- 1 tsp. Worcestershire sauce
- 1-pound crabmeat
- ¼ mug parsley, sliced off
- Table salt and black pepper to the taste
- 2 green onions, sliced off
- 1 tsp. old bay seasoning
- ½ tsp. mustard grinding grains
- ½ mug mayonnaise
- 1 egg
- 2 tbsp olive oil

Instructions:

- In an enormous pot join crab meat with table salt, pepper, parsley, green onions, cilantro, jalapeno, lemon juice, old straight flavoring, mustard crushing grains and Worcestershire sauce and shake well indeed. In another pot join egg mind mayo and whisk. Addition this to crabmeat consolidate and shake everything.
- Shape 6 patties from this join and Put them on a plate. Warm up a dish with the oil over moderate monstrous warmth, embed 3 crab cakes, get ready for 3 minutes, flip, set them up for 3 minutes more and move to paper towels. Rehash with the other 3 crab cakes, channel overabundance oil and serve for lunch.

Lunch Muffin

Ingredients:

- ¾ mug coconut flour
- 1-pound beef, ground
- Table salt to the taste
- 6 egg yolks
- 2 tbsp coconut aminos
- ½ pound mushrooms

Instructions:

- In your food processor, combine mushrooms with table salt, coconut aminos and egg yolks and blend well. In a pot, combine beef meat with some table salt and shake. Insert mushroom combine to beef and shake everything. Insert coconut flour and shake again.
- Distribute this into 13 mug cake mugs, introduce in the oven at 350 degrees f and bake for 45 minutes. Serve them for lunch

Chicken Livers Lunch Pate

Ingredients:

- Table salt and black pepper to the taste
- 3 tbsp butter
- 3 radishes, thinly sliced
- 4 ounces chicken livers, sautéed
- 1 tsp. combined thyme, sage and oregano, sliced off
- Crusted bread slices for serving

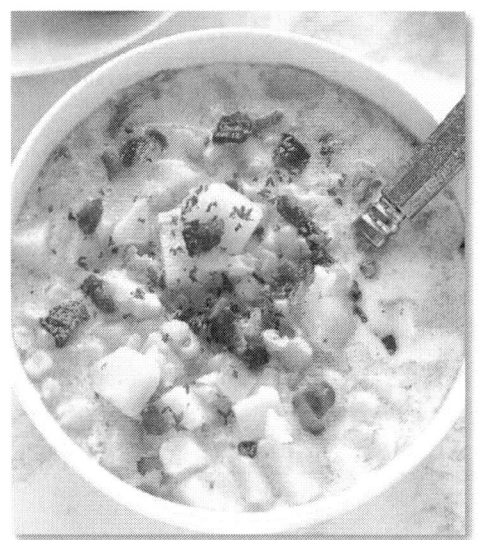

Instructions:

- In your food processor, combine chicken livers with thyme, sage, oregano, butter, table salt and pepper and blend very well for a few minutes. Scatter on crusted bread slices and top with radishes slices. Serve right away.

Delicious Lunch Chowder

Ingredients:

- Juice from 1 lime
- Table salt and black pepper to the taste
- 1 jalapeno pepper, sliced off
- Cheddar cheese, shredded for serving
- Lime wedges for serving
- 1 yellow onion, sliced off
- 1-pound chicken immense, skinless and boneless
- 10 ounces canned tomatoes, sliced off
- 1 mug chicken stock
- 8 ounces cream cheese
- 2 tbsp cilantro, sliced off
- 1 garlic clove, chopped

Instructions:

- In your crock pot, combine chicken with tomatoes, stock, cream cheese, table salt, pepper, lime juice, jalapeno, onion, garlic and cilantro, shake, wrap up and prepare on Immense for 4 hours. Unwrap up pot, shred meat into the pot, distribute into pots and serve with cheddar cheese on top and lime wedges on the side.

Fish Coconut Soup

Ingredients:

- 1 tsp. lemongrass, dried
- 1 mug cilantro, sliced off
- 2 tbsp mushrooms, sliced off

- 1 tablespoon fish sauce
- 1 tablespoon cilantro, sliced off
- Juice from 1 lime
- 1-inch ginger, grated
- 4 Thai chilies, dried and sliced off
- Table salt and black pepper to the taste
- 4 ounces shrimp, raw, peeled and deveined
- 4 mugs chicken stock
- 3 lime leaves
- 1 and ½ mugs coconut milk
- 2 tbsp red onion, sliced off
- 1 tablespoon coconut oil

Instructions:

- In a pot, combine chicken stock with coconut milk, lime leaves, lemongrass, Thai chilies, 1 mug cilantro, ginger, table salt and pepper, shake, bring to a simmer over moderate heat, prepare for 20 minutes, strain and return to pot.
- Warm up soup again over moderate heat, insert coconut oil, shrimp, fish sauce, mushrooms and onions, shake and prepare for 10 minutes more. Insert lime juice and 1 tablespoon cilantro, shake, ladle into pots and serve for lunch

Onion Noodles Soup
Ingredients:

- 1 tablespoon coconut oil
- 1 red bell pepper, sliced
- 2 tbsp fish sauce
- 2 zucchinis, slice with a spiralizer
- 1 and ½ tbsp curry paste
- 6 mugs chicken stock
- 15 ounces canned coconut milk
- 1 small yellow onion, sliced off
- 2 garlic cloves, chopped
- 1 jalapeno pepper, sliced off
- 1-pound chicken breasts, sliced
- ½ mug cilantro, sliced off
- Lime wedges for serving

Instructions:

- Warm up a pot with the oil over moderate heat, insert onion, shake and prepare for 5 minutes. Insert garlic, jalapeno and curry paste, shake and prepare for 1 minute. Insert stock and coconut milk, shake and bring to a boil. Insert red bell pepper, chicken and fish sauce, shake and simmer for 4 minutes more.

- Insert cilantro, shake, prepare for 1 minute and remove heat. Distribute zucchini noodles into soup pots, insert soup on top and serve with lime wedges on the side.

Cinnamon Lunch Curry

Ingredients:

- 2 teaspoons coriander, ground
- 1 tsp. cinnamon, ground
- 1 tsp. turmeric, ground
- 1 tsp. cumin, ground
- 1 tablespoon lime juice
- Table salt and black pepper to the taste
- 2 pounds chicken immense, boneless and skinless and cubed
- 2 garlic cloves, chopped
- 1 mug white onion, sliced off
- 3 red chilies, sliced off
- 3 tomatoes, sliced off
- 2 tbsp olive oil
- 1 mug chicken stock
- 14 ounces canned coconut milk
- 1-ounce peanuts, toasted
- 1 tablespoon water
- 1 tablespoon ginger, grated
- ½ tsp. black pepper
- 1 tsp. fennel seeds, ground

Instructions:

- In your food processor, consolidate white onion with garlic, peanuts, red chilies, water, ginger, coriander, cinnamon, turmeric, cumin, fennel and dark pepper, mix until you acquire a glue and leave aside for the time being.
- Warm up a dish with the olive oil over moderate massive warmth, embed flavor glue you've made, shake well and Warm up for a couple of moments. Addition chicken pieces shake and plan for 2 minutes.
- Addition stock and tomatoes, shake, decrease warmth to low and plan for 30 minutes. Supplement coconut milk, shake and get ready for 20 minutes more. Addition table salt, pepper and lime juice, shake, disseminate into pots and serve.

Parmesan Spinach Rolls

Ingredients:

- A pinch of table salt
- ¼ mug parmesan, grated
- Mayonnaise for serving
- 4 ounces cream cheese

- 6 ounces spinach, torn
- 6 tbsp coconut flour
- ½ mug almond flour
- 2 and ½ mugs mozzarella cheese, shredded
- 2 eggs
- A drizzle of avocado oil
- A pinch of table salt

Instructions:

- Warm up a dish with the oil over moderate warmth, embed spinach and plan for 2 minutes. Addition parmesan, a spot of table salt and cream cheddar, shake well, eliminate warmth and leave aside until further notice.
- Put mozzarella cheddar in a heatproof pot and microwave for 30 seconds. Addition eggs, table salt, coconut and almond flour and shake everything. Put mixture on a lined board, put a material paper on top and straighten batter with a moving pin. Disseminate mixture into 16 square shapes, Scatter spinach join on each and fold them into stogie shapes.
- Put all moves on a lined preparing sheet, present in the broiler at 350 degrees F and heat for 15 minutes. Leave moves to chill off for a couple of moments prior to serving them with some mayo on top.

Avocados Steak Pot
Ingredients:

- Table salt and black pepper to the taste
- 1 handful cilantro, sliced off
- 1 tablespoon cilantro, sliced off
- Table salt and black pepper to the taste
- A splash of chipotle adobo sauce
- ¼ mug red onion, sliced off
- 2 avocados, pitted and peeled
- Juice from 1 lime
- 16 ounces skirt steak
- 4 ounces pepper jack cheese, shredded
- 1 mug sour cream
- 1 tablespoon olive oil
- 6 cherry tomatoes, sliced off
- 1 garlic clove, chopped

Instructions:

- Put avocados in a pot and mash with a fork. Insert tomatoes, red onion, garlic, table salt and pepper and shake well. Insert olive oil, lime juice and 1 tablespoon cilantro, shake again very well and leave aside for now.
- Warm up a dish over immense heat, insert steak, season with table salt and pepper, prepare for 4 minutes on each side, shift to a board, leave aside to cool down a bit and slice into thin

strips. Distribute steak into 4 pots, insert cheese, sour cream and guacamole on top and serve with a splash of chipotle adobo sauce.

Mexican Lunch

Ingredients:

- ¼ mug white onion, sliced off
- 1 tsp. garlic, chopped
- ¼ mug taco seasoning
- 2 mugs lettuce leaves, shredded
- Some cayenne pepper sauce for serving
- 2 mugs cheddar cheese, shredded
- Table salt and black pepper to the taste
- 6 cherry tomatoes, slice in quarters
- ½ mug water
- ¼ mug cilantro, sliced off
- 2 avocados, pitted, peeled and slice into chunks
- 1 tablespoon lime juice
- 2-pound beef meat, ground
- 2 mugs sour cream

Instructions:

- In a pot, combine cilantro with lime juice, avocado, onion, tomatoes, table salt, pepper and garlic, shake well and leave aside in the fridge for now. Warm up a dish over moderate heat, insert beef, shake and brown for 10 minutes. Insert taco seasoning and water, shake and prepare over moderate-low heat for 10 minutes more.
- Distribute this combine into 4 serving pots. Insert sour cream, avocado combine you've made earlier, lettuce pieces and cheddar cheese. Drizzle cayenne pepper sauce at the end and serve for lunch

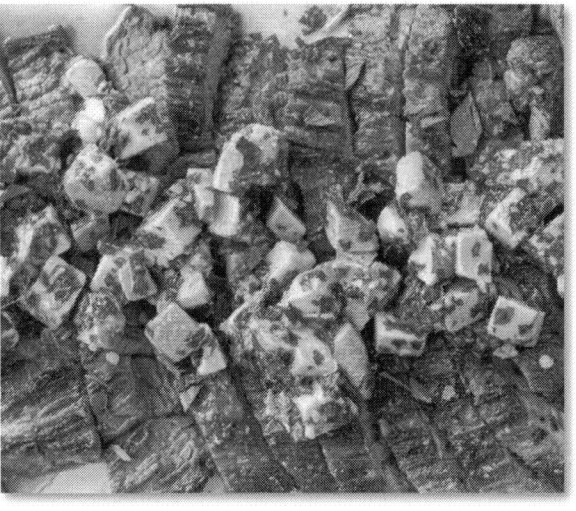

Meatballs, Paprika and Pilaf

Ingredients:

- 1 tsp. fennel seed
- 1 tsp. paprika
- 1 tsp. garlic grinding grains
- 1 tablespoon lemon zest
- 4 ounces goat cheese, crumbled
- 1 small yellow onion, sliced off
- 2 garlic cloves, chopped
- 12 ounces cauliflower florets

- Table salt and black pepper to the taste
- 1 egg
- 1-pound lamb, ground
- 2 tbsp coconut oil
- 1 bunch mint, sliced off

Instructions:

- Put cauliflower florets in your food processor, embed table salt and heartbeat well. Oil a dish with a portion of the coconut oil, Warm up over moderate warmth, embed cauliflower rice, plan for 8 minutes, season with table salt and pepper to the taste, eliminate warmth and keep warm. In a pot, consolidate sheep with table salt, pepper, egg, paprika, garlic crushing grains and fennel seed and shake well indeed.
- Shape 12 meatballs and Put them on a plate until further notice. Warm up a dish with the coconut oil over moderate warmth, embed onion, shake and get ready for 6 minutes.
- Supplement garlic, shake and get ready for 1 moment. Addition meatballs set them up well on all sides and eliminate heat. Disperse cauliflower rice between plates, embed meatballs and onion join on top, Garnish mint, lemon zing and goat cheddar toward the end and serve.

Broccoli Soup

Ingredients:

- Table salt and black pepper to the taste
- 2 mugs water
- 12 ounces broccoli florets
- ½ tsp. paprika
- 2 garlic cloves, chopped
- 1 white onion, sliced off
- 1 tablespoon ghee
- 2 mugs veggie stock
- 1 mug heavy cream
- 8 ounces cheddar cheese, grated

Instructions:

- Warm up a pot with the ghee over moderate heat, insert onion and garlic, shake and prepare for 5 minutes. Insert stock, cream, water, table salt, pepper and paprika, shake and bring to a boil. Insert broccoli, shake and simmer soup for 25 minutes.
- Shift to your food processor and blend well. Insert cheese and blend again. Distribute into soup pots and serve warm.

Green Beans Salad

Ingredients:

- Table salt and black pepper to the taste
- 2 pounds green beans

- 4 ounces goat cheese, crumbled
- ¾ mug walnuts, toasted and sliced off
- 1/3 mug extra virgin olive oil
- 2 tbsp white wine vinegar
- 1 and ½ tbsp mustard
- 1 and ½ mugs fennel, thinly sliced

Instructions:

- Put water in a pot, insert some table salt and bring to a boil over moderate immense heat. Insert green beans, prepare for 5 minutes and shift them to a pot filled with ice water. Drain green beans well and put them in a salad pot.
- Insert walnuts, fennel and goat cheese and fling gently. In a pot, combine vinegar with mustard, table salt, pepper and oil and whisk well. Pour this over salad, fling to coat well and serve for lunch.

Creamy Pumpkin Soup
Ingredients:

- 1 garlic clove, chopped
- 1 tsp. cumin, ground
- 1 tsp. coriander, ground
- A pinch of allspice
- ½ mug heavy cream
- 2 teaspoons vinegar
- 2 teaspoons stevia
- ½ mug yellow onion, sliced off
- 2 tbsp olive oil
- 1 tablespoon chipotles in adobo sauce
- 2 mugs pumpkin puree
- Table salt and black pepper to the taste

32 ounces chicken stock

Instructions:

- Warm up a pot with the oil over moderate heat, insert onions and garlic, shake and prepare for 4 minutes. Insert stevia, cumin, coriander, chipotles and cumin, shake and prepare for 2 minutes. Insert stock and pumpkin puree, shake and prepare for 5 minutes.
- Blend soup well using an immersion blender and then combine with table salt, pepper, heavy cream and vinegar. Shake, prepare for 5 minutes more and Distribute into pots. Serve right away.

Green Beans Casserole
Ingredients:

- 2 tbsp ghee
- 8 ounces mushrooms, sliced off

- 4 ounces onion, sliced off
- 2 shallots, sliced off
- ½ mug heavy cream
- ¼ mug parmesan, grated
- Avocado oil for frying
- 3 garlic cloves, chopped
- 1-pound green beans, halved
- Table salt and black pepper to the taste
- ½ mug almond flour
- ½ mug chicken stock

Instructions:

- Put some water in a pot, embed table salt, heat to the point of boiling over moderate tremendous warmth, embed green beans, plan for 5 minutes, move to a pot loaded up with ice water, chill off, channel well and leave aside until further notice.
- In a pot, consolidate shallots with onions, almond flour, table salt and pepper and throw to cover. Warm up a dish with some avocado oil over moderate colossal warmth, embed onions and shallots join, fry until they are brilliant.
- Move to paper towels and channel oil. Warm up a similar dish over moderate warmth, embed ghee and soften it. Supplement garlic and mushrooms shake and plan for 5 minutes. Addition stock and hefty cream, shake, heat to the point of boiling and stew until it thickens.
- Addition parmesan and green beans throw to cover and eliminate heat. Move this consolidate to a heating dish, Garnish firm onions join all finished, present in the stove at 400 degrees F and prepare for 15 minutes. Serve warm.

Lunch Apple Salad

Ingredients:

- 1 green onion stalk, finely sliced off
- ½ tsp. lemon juice
- ¼ mug sour cream
- Table salt and black pepper to the taste
- 2 teaspoons poppy seeds
- 1 tsp. apple cider vinegar
- 2 mugs broccoli florets, roughly sliced off
- 2 ounces pecans, sliced off
- 1 apple, cored and grated
- ¼ mug mayonnaise

Instructions:

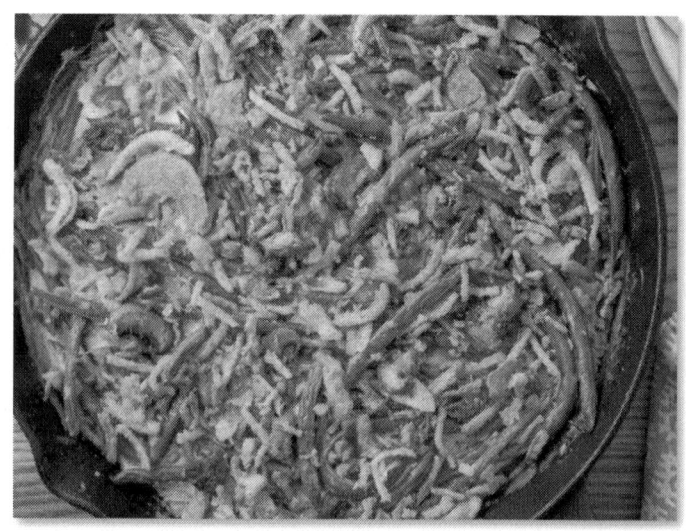

- In a salad pot, combine apple with broccoli, green onion and pecans and shake. Insert poppy seeds, table salt and pepper and fling gently.

- In a pot, combine mayo with sour cream, vinegar and lemon juice and whisk well. Pour this over salad, fling to coat well and serve cold for lunch

Brussels Sprouts Gratin

Ingredients:

- 2 tbsp ghee
- ¼ tsp. turmeric
- ¼ tsp. paprika
- A pinch of xanthan gum
- 3 tbsp parmesan
- 1 tablespoon coconut aminos
- Table salt and black pepper to the taste
- ½ tsp. liquid smoke
- 2 ounces onions, sliced off
- 1 tsp. garlic, chopped
- 6 ounces Brussels sprouts, sliced off
- 2.5 ounces cheddar cheese, grated
- A pinch of black pepper
- 1 tablespoon ghee
- ½ mug heavy cream
- 0.5 ounces pork rinds
- ½ tsp. sweet paprika

Instructions:

- Heat the plate with 2 tablespoons of ghee over high heat, add Brussels sprouts, salt and pepper, beat and cook for 3 minutes. Add the garlic and onions, beat and cook for 3 more minutes. Add liquid smoke and coconut amino acids, shake, remove heat and set aside first. Heat other dishes with 1 tablespoon of melted butter over medium heat, add cream and beat. Add cheese, black pepper, turmeric, paprika and xanthan gum, beat and cook until thickened again. Add Brussels sprouts, stir, cover and spread on a baking sheet.
- Combine parmesan with pork skin and ½ teaspoon in your food processor. Peppers and veins are good. Spread these crumbs over the combined Brussels sprouts, place the casserole dish in the oven at 375 degrees F, and bake for 20 minutes. Serve immediately.

Egg Asparagus Lunch

Ingredients:

- ¼ mug ghee
- 1 tablespoon lemon juice
- 2 egg yolks
- Table salt and black pepper to the taste
- A pinch of cayenne pepper
- 40 asparagus spears

Instructions:

- In a pot, whisk egg yolks very well. Shift this to a small dish over low heat. Insert lemon juice and whisk well. Insert ghee and whisk until it melts. Insert table salt, pepper and cayenne pepper and whisk again well.
- Meanwhile, Warm up a dish over moderate immense heat, insert asparagus spears and fry them for 5 minutes. Distribute asparagus on plates, drizzle the sauce you've made on top and serve.

Mexican Casserole

Ingredients:

- ¼ mug heavy cream
- 1 small white onion, sliced off
- Table salt and black pepper to the taste
- 2 chipotle peppers, sliced off
- 2 jalapenos, sliced off
- 1 tablespoon olive oil
- 1-pound chicken immense, skinless, boneless and sliced off
- 1 mug pepper jack cheese, shredded
- 2 tbsp cilantro, sliced off
- 2 tortillas
- 1 mug red enchilada sauce
- 4 ounces cream cheese
- Preparing spray

Instructions:

- Heat the plate with 2 tablespoons of ghee over high heat, add Brussels sprouts, salt and pepper, beat and cook for 3 minutes. Add the garlic and onions, beat and cook for 3 more minutes. Add liquid smoke and coconut amino acids, shake, remove heat and set aside first. Heat other dishes with 1 tablespoon of melted butter over medium heat, add cream and beat. Add cheese, black pepper, turmeric, paprika and xanthan gum, beat and cook until thickened again. Add Brussels sprouts, stir, cover and spread on a baking sheet. Combine parmesan with pork skin and ½ teaspoon in your food processor.
- Peppers and veins are good. Spread these crumbs over the combined Brussels sprouts, place the casserole dish in the oven at 375 degrees F, and bake for 20 minutes. Serve immediately.

Green Asian Lunch Salad

Ingredients:

- 2 garlic cloves, chopped
- 10 ounces coleslaw combine
- 1 tsp. sesame seeds
- 1 green onion stalk, sliced off
- 2 tablespoon sesame seed oil

- Table salt and black pepper to the taste
- 1-pound beef, ground
- 1 tablespoon sriracha
- 2 tbsp coconut aminos
- 1 tsp. apple cider vinegar

Instructions:

- Warm up a dish with the oil over moderate heat, insert garlic and brown for 1 minute. Insert beef, shake and prepare for 10 minutes.
- Insert Cole slaw combine, fling to coat and prepare for 1minute. Insert vinegar, sriracha, coconut aminos, table salt and pepper, shake and prepare for 4 minutes more. Insert green onions and sesame seeds, fling to coat, distribute into pots and serve for lunch.

Masala Buffalo Wings
Ingredients:

- Table salt and black pepper to the taste
- A pinch of garlic grinding grains
- ½ mug warm sauce
- A pinch of cayenne pepper
- 2 tbsp ghee
- 6 chicken wings, slice in halves
- ½ tsp. sweet paprika

Instructions:

- In a pot, combine chicken pieces with half of the warm sauce, table salt and pepper and fling well to coat. Organize chicken pieces on a lined baking dish, introduce in preheated broiler and broil 8 minutes. Flip chicken pieces and broil for 8 minutes more. Warm up a dish with the ghee over moderate heat. Insert the rest of the warm sauce, table salt, pepper, cayenne and paprika, shake and prepare for a couple of minutes.
- Shift broiled chicken pieces to a pot, insert ghee and warm sauce combine over them and fling to coat well. Serve them right away.

Bacon and Mushrooms Skewers
Ingredients:

- Table salt and black pepper to the taste
- ½ tsp. sweet paprika
- 1-pound mushroom caps
- 6 bacon strips
- Some sweet mesquites

Instructions:

- Season mushroom caps with table salt, pepper and paprika. Spear a bacon strip on a skewer's ends. Spear a mushroom cap and fold over bacon.
- Repeat until you obtain a mushroom and bacon braid. Repeat with the rest of the mushrooms and bacon strip. Season with sweet mesquite, put all skewers on preheated kitchen grill over moderate heat, prepare for 10 minutes, flip and prepare for 10 minutes more. Distribute between plates and serve for lunch with a side salad.

Green Soup
Ingredients:

- 2 garlic cloves, chopped
- 5 ounces watercress
- 7 ounces spinach leaves
- 1-quart veggie stock
- 1 mug coconut milk
- 1 cauliflower head, florets separated
- 1 white onion, finely sliced off
- 1 bay leaf, crushed
- Table salt and black pepper to the taste
- ¼ mug ghee
- A handful parsley, for serving

Instructions:

- Warm up a pot with the ghee over moderate immense heat, insert garlic and onion, shake and brown for 4 minutes. Insert cauliflower and bay leaf, shake and prepare for 5 minutes. Insert watercress and spinach, shake and prepare for 3 minutes.
- Insert stock, table salt and pepper, shake and bring to a boil. Insert coconut milk, shake, remove heat and blend using an immersion blender. Distribute into pots and serve right away.

Tomato Soup
Ingredients:

- 2 tbsp apple cider vinegar
- Table salt and black pepper to the taste
- 1 tsp. oregano, dried
- 2 tsp. turmeric, ground
- 1-quart canned tomato soup
- 4 tbsp ghee
- ¼ mug olive oil
- ¼ mug red warm sauce
- 8 bacon strips, prepared and crumbled
- A handful green onions, sliced off

- A handful basil leaves, sliced off

Instructions:

- Put tomato soup in a pot and Warm up over moderate heat. Insert olive oil, ghee, warm sauce, vinegar, table salt, pepper, turmeric and oregano, shake and simmer for 5 minutes. Remove heat, Distribute soup into pots, top with bacon crumbles, basil and green onions.

Bacon Wrapped Sausages
Ingredients:

- Table salt and black pepper to the taste
- A pinch of garlic grinding grains
- ½ tsp. sweet paprika
- 8 bacon strips
- 8 sausages
- 16 pepper jack cheese slices
- 1 pinch of onion grinding grains

Instructions:

- Warm up your kitchen grill over moderate heat, insert sausages, prepare for a few minutes on each side, shift to a plate and leave them aside for a few minutes to cool down. Slice a slit in the middle of each sausage to create pockets, stuff each with 2 cheese slices and season with table salt, pepper, paprika, onion and garlic grinding grains.
- Wrap each stuffed sausage in a bacon strip, secure with toothpicks, put on a lined baking sheet, introduce in the oven at 400 degrees F and bake for 15 minutes. Serve warm for lunch

Cloves Lobster Bisque
Ingredients:

- Table salt and black pepper to the taste
- ½ mug tomato paste
- 2 carrots, finely sliced off
- 4 celery stalks, sliced off
- 4 garlic cloves, chopped
- 1 small red onion, sliced off
- 24 ounces lobster chunks, pre-prepared
- 1-quart seafood stock
- 1 tablespoon olive oil
- 1 tsp. peppercorns
- 1 tsp. paprika
- 1 tsp. xanthan gum
- A handful parsley, sliced off
- 1 mug heavy cream
- 3 bay leaves

- 1 tsp. thyme, dried
- 1 tablespoon lemon juice

Instructions:

- Warm up a pot with the oil over moderate heat, insert onion, shake and prepare for 4 minutes. Insert garlic, shake and prepare for 1 minute more.
- Insert celery and carrot, shake and prepare for 1 minute. Insert tomato paste and stock and shake everything. Insert bay leaves, table salt, pepper, peppercorns, paprika, thyme and xanthan gum, shake and simmer over moderate heat for 1 hour. Remove bay leaves, insert cream and bring to a simmer. Blend using an immersion blender, insert lobster chunks and prepare for a few minutes more. Insert lemon juice, shake, Distribute into pots and Garnish parsley on top.

Green Halloumi Salad
Ingredients:

- A handful baby arugula
- 5 cherry tomatoes, halved
- A splash of balsamic vinegar
- 3 ounces halloumi cheese, sliced
- 1 cucumber, sliced
- 1-ounce walnuts, sliced off
- A drizzle of olive oil
- Table salt and black pepper to the taste

Instructions:

- Warm up your kitchen grill over moderate immense heat, insert halloumi pieces, grill them for 5 minutes on each side and shift to a plate.
- In a pot, combine tomatoes with cucumber, walnuts and arugula. Insert halloumi pieces on top, season everything with table salt, pepper, drizzle the oil and the vinegar, fling to coat and serve.

Lunch Vegetables Stew
Ingredients:

- 2 onions, sliced off
- 2 mugs water
- 1-quart chicken stock
- ¼ mug tomato sauce
- 2 teaspoons parsley, dried
- 2 teaspoons basil, dried
- 2 teaspoons garlic grinding grains
- 2 teaspoons onion grinding grains
- Table salt and black pepper to the taste

- 2 tbsp apple cider vinegar
- 8 tomatoes, sliced off
- 5 pounds beef shanks
- 3 carrots, sliced off
- 8 garlic cloves, chopped
- 3 bay leaves
- 3 teaspoons red pepper, crushed
- A pinch of cayenne pepper

Instructions:

- Heat the pan over medium heat, add the garlic, carrots and onions, beat and brown for a few minutes. Heat a skillet over medium heat, brown the thighs on each side for a few minutes, then turn off the heat.
- Pour the carrots, water and vinegar, then beat. Add the tomato, ketchup, salt, pepper, cayenne pepper, ground pepper, bay leaf, basil, parsley, onion grinder and garlic grinder and beat everything. Enter the beef thighs, wrap the pan, bring to a boil and cook for 3 hours. Remove the bay leaves, arrange in a pot and serve.

Shrimp and Chicken

Ingredients:

- ½ pound mushrooms, roughly sliced off
- Table salt and black pepper to the taste
- ¼ mug mayonnaise
- 2 tbsp sriracha
- ½ tsp. paprika
- ¼ tsp. xanthan gum
- 1 green onion stalk, sliced off
- 20 shrimp, raw, peeled and deveined
- 2 chicken breasts, boneless and skinless
- 2 handfuls spinach leaves
- 2 teaspoons lime juice
- 1 tablespoon coconut oil
- ½ tsp. red pepper, crushed
- 1 tsp. garlic grinding grains

Instructions:

- Warm up a dish with the oil over moderate gigantic warmth, embed chicken bosoms, season with table salt, pepper, red pepper and garlic pounding grains, plan for 8 minutes, flip and get ready for 6 minutes more. Supplement mushrooms, more table salt and pepper and plan for a couple of moments.
- Warm up another dish over moderate warmth, embed shrimp, sriracha, paprika, xanthan and mayo, shake and get ready until shrimp turn pink. Eliminate heat, embed lime squeeze and shake everything.

- Convey spinach on plates, appropriate chicken and mushroom, top with shrimp consolidate, decorate with green onions and serve.

Salmon Soup

Ingredients:

- 2 garlic cloves, chopped
- 6 mugs chicken stock
- 1-pound salmon, slice into small pieces
- 2 teaspoons thyme, dried
- 4 leeks, trimmed and sliced
- Table salt and black pepper to the taste
- 2 tbsp avocado oil
- 1 and ¾ mugs coconut milk

Instructions:

- Warm up a pot with the oil over moderate heat, insert leeks and garlic, shake and prepare for 5 minutes. Insert thyme, stock, table salt and pepper, shake and simmer for 15 minutes. Insert coconut milk and salmon, shake and bring to a simmer again. Distribute into pots and serve right away.

Halibut Soup

Ingredients:

- Table salt and black pepper to the taste
- 2 tbsp ginger, chopped
- 1 mug water
- 1 yellow onion, sliced off
- 1-pound carrots, sliced
- 1 tablespoon coconut oil
- 1-pound halibut, slice into moderate chunks
- 12 mugs chicken stock

Instructions:

- Warm up a pot with the oil over moderate heat, insert onion, shake and prepare for 6 minutes. Insert ginger, carrots, water and stock, shake bring to a simmer, reduce tempera and prepare for 20 minutes.
- Blend soup using an immersion blender, season with table salt and pepper and insert halibut pieces. Shake gently and simmer soup for 5 minutes more. Distribute into pots and serve.

Dijon-Style Mustard Cherry-Sage Scotch Eggs

Ingredients:

- 1 tablespoon snipped fresh marjoram
- 1 tsp. freshly ground black pepper
- ½ tsp. dried marjoram, crushed
- 2 tbsp extra virgin olive oil
- Dijon-Style Mustard
- ¼ tsp. freshly ground nutmeg
- ⅛ tsp. ground cloves
- 1-pound lean ground pork
- ½ mug snipped no-sugar-inserted dried cherries
- 2 tbsp snipped fresh sage
- 4 hard-prepared large eggs, cooled and peeled
- ½ mug almond flour
- 1 tsp. dried sage, crushed

Instructions:

- Preheat broiler to 375°F. Line a heating dish with material paper or foil; put in a safe spot. In an enormous pot join pork, cherries, new wise, new marjoram, pepper, nutmeg, and cloves. Shape pork consolidate into four equivalent patties. Put one egg on every patty. Shape the patty around each egg. In a shallow dish or pie plate join almond flour, dried sage, and dried marjoram.
- Roll every wiener covered egg in the almond flour join to cover. Put on the readied heating sheet. Shower with olive oil. Heat for 35 to 40 minutes or until hotdog is set up through. Present with Dijon-Style Mustard.

Cauliflower Eggs and Steaks

Ingredients:

- 5 tbsp extra virgin olive oil
- 4 large eggs
- 1 tablespoon white or cider vinegar
- 2 large cloves garlic, chopped
- 1 head cauliflower, leaves removed
- 1½ teaspoons Smoky Seasoning
- 4 mugs sliced off kale

Instructions:

- Put stem finish of cauliflower on a   board. Using a large sharp knife, slice cauliflower into four ½-inch steaks from the center of the cauliflower, through stem end (some florets could break loose; save for another use). Season steaks on each side with one tsp. of the Smoky Seasoning. In a further-giant skillet heat two tbsp of the olive oil over moderate-immense heat. Insert two of the cauliflower steaks. Prepare for 4 minutes on every side or till golden brown and simply tender.

- Remove from dish and Wrap up lightly with foil. Keep warm in a 200°F oven. Repeat with remaining 2 steaks, using a 2 tbsp of olive oil. To poach the eggs, fill a separate skillet with concerning 3 inches of water. Insert vinegar and produce to a simmer. Crack eggs, one by one, into a small pot or ramekin and gently slide into the simmering water. Let eggs prepare for 30 to forty-five seconds or till whites begin to firm up.
- Turn off the heat. Wrap up and poach for 3 to five minutes, relying on how soft you prefer your yolks. Meanwhile, in the same skillet heat the remaining 1 tablespoon olive oil. Insert garlic and prepare for thirty seconds to one minute. Insert kale and prepare and shake for one to two minutes or just until wilted. To serve, Distribute kale among four plates. Top each with a cauliflower steak and a poached egg. Garnish eggs with the remaining ½ tsp. Smoky Seasoning and serve.

Turkey and Asparagus Frittata

Ingredients:

- ¼ to ½ tsp. black pepper
- ½ mug ½-inch-long pieces fresh asparagus
- 1 mug fresh baby spinach leaves, sliced off
- 4 large eggs
- 1 tablespoon water
- 2 tbsp extra virgin olive oil
- 1 clove garlic, chopped
- 4 ounces ground turkey breast
- 2 teaspoons snipped fresh dill
- 1 tablespoon snipped fresh parsley

Instructions:

- Preheat broiler with the oven rack positioned four inches from the heating element. In an oven-safe moderate skillet heat one tablespoon of the olive oil over moderate heat. Insert garlic; prepare and shake until golden. Insert the bottom turkey, Garnish with pepper. Prepare and shake for 3 to 4 minutes or till meat is browned and prepared through, shake ring with a picket spoon to break up meat.
- Shift ready turkey to a pot; set aside. Return skillet to stovetop; pour the remaining 1 tablespoon olive oil into skillet. Insert asparagus; prepare and shake over moderate-immense heat till tender.
- Shake in the prepared turkey and therefore the spinach. Prepare for one minute. In a moderate pot beat eggs with the water and the dill. Pour egg combine over turkey mix in skillet. Prepare and shake for 1 minute. Shift skillet to oven and broil for 3 to 4 minutes or till eggs are set and prime is browned. Garnish with snipped parsley.

Parsley Scrambled Eggs and Harissa

Ingredients:

- 6 large eggs
- ¼ tsp. ground cinnamon
- ½ tsp. ground cumin
- ⅓ mug golden raisins
- ⅓ mug snipped fresh parsley
- 1 small red sweet pepper
- 1 small yellow sweet pepper
- 1 small poblano chile pepper
- 1 tablespoon extra-virgin olive oil
- 1 tablespoon Harissa

Instructions:

- Preheat broiler with the oven rack positioned 3 to 4 inches from the heat. Halve peppers lengthwise; remove stems and seeds. Place pepper halves, slice sides down, on a foil-lined baking sheet. Broil eight minutes or until pepper skins are black.
- Wrap peppers in the foil. Let cool for five minutes. Unwrap peppers; use a sharp knife to peel away blackened skins. Slice peppers into skinny strips; set aside. In a giant pot combine eggs, cinnamon, and cumin.
- Whisk until frothy. Insert pepper strips, raisins, parsley, and Harissa. In a massive skillet heat olive oil over moderate heat. Insert the egg mix to skillet. Prepare regarding 5 to 7 minutes or till eggs are set however still moist and shiny, shake ring frequently. Serve instantly.

Fresh Basil Eggs Shakshuka

Ingredients:

- 1 tsp. ground cumin
- ½ tsp. smoked paprika
- ½ tsp. crushed red pepper
- 4 cloves garlic, chopped
- ¼ mug extra virgin olive oil
- 1 large onion, halved and thinly sliced
- 1 large red sweet pepper, thinly sliced
- 1 large orange sweet pepper, thinly sliced
- 2 14.5-ounce cans organic table salt-free fire-roasted diced tomatoes
- 6 large eggs
- Freshly ground black pepper
- ¼ mug snipped fresh cilantro
- ¼ mug shredded fresh basil

Instructions:

- Preheat oven to four hundred °F. In an oven-safe giant skillet heat oil over moderate heat. Insert onion and sweet peppers. Prepare and shake for four to five minutes or till vegetables are tender. Insert cumin, paprika, crushed red pepper, and garlic; prepare and shake for two minutes. Shake in tomatoes.
- Bring to boiling; cut back heat. Simmer, unwrap upped, about ten minutes or till thickened. Crack eggs into skillet over tomato mix. Shift skillet to the preheated oven. Bake, unwrap upped, for seven to ten minutes or till eggs are simply set (yolks should still be runny). Garnish with black pepper. Garnish with cilantro and basil; serve instantly.

Olive Baked Eggs with Salmon

Ingredients:

- 10 ounces baby spinach leaves (6 mugs packed)
- 2 tbsp water
- 8 ounces grilled or roasted salmon
- 1 tsp. finely shredded lemon peel
- 1 tablespoon extra-virgin olive oil
- 1 tablespoon fresh thyme leaves
- Freshly grated nutmeg
- ½ tsp. Smoky Seasoning
- 8 large eggs

Instructions:

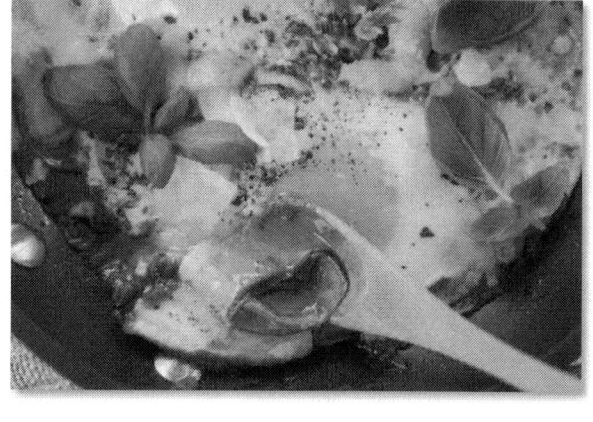

- Preheat oven to 375°F. Brush the insides of 4 six- to eight-ounce ramekins with olive oil. Garnish thyme leaves evenly among the ramekins; gently Garnish with freshly grated nutmeg. Set aside. In a Wrap upped moderate sauce dish mix spinach and also the water. Bring to boiling; take away from heat. Lift and flip spinach with tongs just till wilted. Put spinach in a very fine-mesh sieve; press firmly to release excess liquid.
- Distribute spinach among prepared ramekins. Flake salmon evenly among ramekins.
- Garnish salmon with lemon peel and Smoky Seasoning. Crack two of the eggs into every ramekin. Put filled ramekins in a large baking dish. Pour warm water into the baking dish till it is halfway up the perimeters of the ramekins.
- Carefully shift baking dish to the oven. Bake for fifteen to 18 minutes or until egg whites are set. Serve instantly.

Egg Soup with Scallions and Bok Choy

Ingredients:

- 1 2-inch piece fresh ginger, peeled and slice into very thin matchstick-size strips
- 1-star anise

- 1-pound shiitake mushrooms, stemmed and sliced
- 1 tsp. five-spice grinding grains
- ¼ mug fresh lemon juice
- 3 large eggs
- 6 scallions, thinly sliced
- 2 heads baby book choy, slice into ¼-inch-thick slices
- 0.5-ounce sun-dried wakame
- 3 tbsp unrefined coconut oil
- 2 shallots, chopped
- ¼ tsp. black pepper
- 8 mugs Beef Bone Broth

Instructions:

- In a very moderate pot Wrap up wakame with warm water. Let indicate 10 minutes or till soft and pliable. Drain well; rinse well and drain again. Slice strips of wakame into 1-inch items; put aside. In a very large pot heat coconut oil over moderate heat. Insert shallots, ginger, and star anise.
- Prepare and shake for regarding a pair of minutes or till shallots are translucent. Insert mushrooms; prepare and shake for two minutes.
- Garnish 5-spice grinding grains and pepper over mushrooms; prepare and shake for one minute. Insert reserved wakame, Beef Bone Broth, and lemon juice. Bring combine to simmering. In an exceedingly little pot beat egg. Drizzle overwhelmed eggs into simmering broth, swirling broth in an exceedingly figure-eight motion. Remove soup from heat. Shake in scallions. Distribute book choy among large, warmed pots. Ladle soup into pots; serve instantly.

Snow Crab Meat and Crab

Ingredients:

- ⅓ mug small, diced zucchini
- 1½ ounces fresh or frozen Dungeness or snow crab meat
- 1 1-inch piece fresh ginger, peeled and thinly sliced
- ⅛ tsp. table salt-free five-spice grinding grains
- 3 large eggs, beaten
- 2½ mugs Chicken Bone Broth or notable salt-inserted chicken or beef broth, cooled
- ⅔ mug shiitake mushrooms, stemmed and sliced off
- 2 tbsp snipped fresh cilantro

Instructions:

- Defrost shrimp and crab, whenever frozen. Flush shrimp and crab; wipe off with paper towels. Put in a safe spot. In a little sauce dish bring 1½ mugs stock, ⅓ mug cut off shiitake mushrooms, ginger, and five-zest pounding grains to bubbling; lessen heat. Bubble delicately until diminished to 1 mug, around 15 minutes.

- Eliminate sauce dish from heat. Shake in the leftover 1 cup of stock; let cool to room gum-based paint, around 20 minutes. At the point when stock is cooled totally, delicately race in the eggs, fusing as meager air as could reasonably be expected. Over a pot strain the consolidate through a fine-network sifter; eliminate solids. Appropriate the shrimp, crab, zucchini, cilantro, and the leftover ⅓ mug mushrooms among four 8-to 10-ounce ramekins or mugs. Convey the egg join among the ramekins filling every one-half to three-fourths full; put in a safe spot. Fill an extra-huge stockpot with 1½ crawls of water.

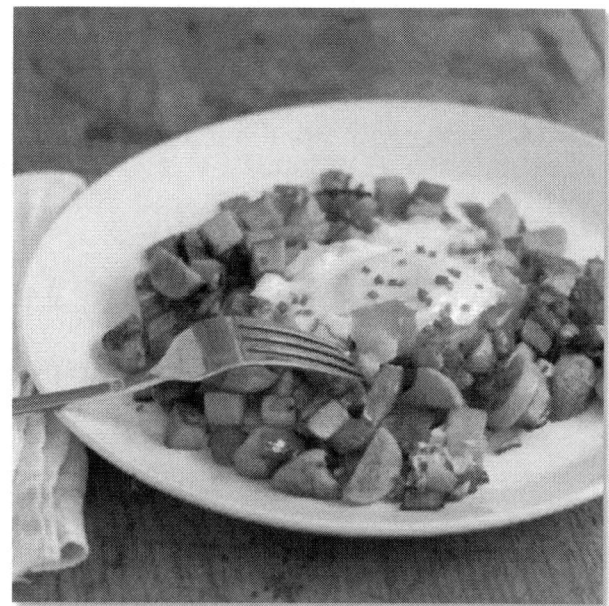

- Wrap up and bring to bubbling. Diminish warmth to direct low. Sort out the four ramekins within the stockpot. Cautiously pour in enough insertional bubbling water to arrive at mostly up the sides of the ramekins.
- Wrap up ramekins freely with foil. Wrap up the pot with a tight-fitting cover and steam around 15 minutes or until egg consolidate is set. To test for doneness, embed a toothpick into the focal point of the custard. At the point when get stock comes out, it is finished. Cautiously eliminate the ramekins. Let cool for 10 minutes prior to serving. Serve warm or cooled.

Chicken Sausage Hash

Ingredients:

- ½ tsp. dried rosemary
- ¼ tsp. black pepper
- 1 mug shredded red or golden beets
- ½ mug Chicken Bone Broth
- 2 tbsp extra virgin olive oil
- 2 mugs sliced off onions
- 2 pounds ground chicken
- 1 tsp. dried thyme
- 1 tsp. dried sage
- 1 tablespoon chopped garlic
- 1 mug sliced off green sweet pepper

Instructions:

- In a large pot combine ground chicken, thyme, sage, rosemary, and black pepper, working combine   together with your hands to evenly distribute seasonings through the meat. In an extra-large skillet heat 1 tablespoon of the oil over moderate-immense heat. Insert chicken; prepare about 8 minutes or until lightly browned, shake ring with a wooden spoon to break up meat.
- Using a slotted spoon, remove meat from skillet; set aside. Drain fat from skillet. Wipe skillet with a clean paper towel. In the same skillet heat the remaining 1 tablespoon oil over moderate heat. Insert onions and garlic; prepare about 3 minutes or until onions are tender.

Insert sweet pepper and shredded beets to onion combine; prepare about 4 to 5 minutes or until vegetables are tender, shake ring occasionally. Shake in reserved chicken combine and Chicken Bone Broth. Heat through.

Carrot Onion Soup with Garam Masala

Ingredients:

- 2 yellow onions, slice into 1½-inch pieces
- 2 tbsp olive oil
- 1 tsp. curry grinding grains
- ¼ tsp. black pepper
- 1 tablespoon grated fresh ginger
- pounds carrots, peeled, if desired, and slice into 1½-inch pieces
- 1½ pounds parsnips, peeled and slice into 1½-inch pieces
- Chicken Bone Broth, notable salt-inserted chicken broth, water, or unsweetened coconut milk (optional)
- Garam Masala Nut "Croutons"
- 2 Granny Smith apples, peeled and slice into 1½-inch pieces
- 6 mugs Chicken Bone Broth
- 1 tsp. ground cumin

Instructions:

- Preheat the broiler to 400°F. Brush an extra-huge, rimmed heating sheet with olive oil. In an extra-enormous pot join carrots, parsnips, apples, and onions. In a little pot consolidate the 2 tbsp olive oil, ½ tsp. of the curry crushing grains, and pepper.
- Pour over vegetables and apples; toss to cover. Disperse vegetables and apples in a solitary layer on the readied heating sheet. Cook for 30 to 40 minutes or until vegetables and apples are delicate. Working in three clumps, put 33% of the vegetable-apple consolidate and the entirety of the ginger in a food processor or blender; embed 2 cups of the Chicken Bone Broth.
- Wrap up and measure until smooth; move to a huge sauce dish. Rehash with staying vegetable-apple consolidate and 4 additional cups of the stock. Addition the leftover ½ tsp. curry granulating grains and the cumin to the pureed join.
- Bring to bubbling; lessen heat. Stew opens up increased, for 10 minutes to merge the flavors. In the event that the soup is excessively thick, slight with insertional stock, water, or coconut milk. Embellishment each presenting with 1 tablespoon of the Garam Masala Nut "Bread garnishes.

Pear Rosemary Sausages

Ingredients:

- 2 teaspoons snipped fresh rosemary
- 1 tsp. fennel seeds, crushed
- ½ tsp. smoked paprika

- ¼ to ½ tsp. freshly ground black pepper
- 1-pound ground pork
- 1 ripe moderate pear (such as Bosc, Anjou, or Bartlett), peeled, cored, and shredded
- 2 tbsp finely sliced off scallions
- 2 cloves garlic, chopped
- 1 tablespoon olive oil

Instructions:

- In a moderate pot mix ground pork, pear, scallions, rosemary, fennel seeds, smoked paprika, pepper, and garlic. Gently mix ingredients till totally combined. Distribute the mix into eight equal parts. Shape into eight ½-inch-thick patties.
- In an extra-large skillet heat olive oil over moderate heat until heat. Insert 0.5 of the patties; prepare for 8 to ten minutes or till well browned and ready through, flipping sausages halfway through. Remove from skillet and Put on a paper towel-lined plate to drain; tent gently with foil to keep heat whereas preparing remaining sausages.

Shredded -Style Shredded Beef

Ingredients:

- 2 teaspoons dried oregano
- ½ tsp. ground cumin
- ½ tsp. ground coriander
- ⅓ mug fresh orange juice
- 1 mug halved cherry tomatoes
- 1 tablespoon fresh lime juice
- ½ tsp. smoked paprika
- 3 cloves garlic, chopped
- 1 bunch collard greens or 4 mugs lightly packed raw spinach
- 2 tbsp extra virgin olive oil
- ½ mug sliced off onion
- 2 moderate green sweet peppers, slice into strips
- 2 ounces prepared beef, shredded
- 1 tsp. finely shredded orange peel
- 1 ripe avocado, seeded, peeled, and sliced

Instructions:

- Remove and take away thick stems from collard greens. Slice leaves into bite-size items; put aside. In a further-giant skillet heat olive oil over moderate heat. Insert onion and sweet peppers; prepare for 3 to 5 minutes or just till vegetables are tender. Insert oregano, cumin, coriander, smoked paprika, and garlic; shake well.
- Insert shredded beef, orange peel, and orange juice; shake to mix. Insert collard greens and tomatoes. Prepare, wrap upped, for 5 minutes or just till tomatoes begin to juice out and collard greens are just tender. Drizzle with lime juice. Serve with sliced avocado.

Asian Poulet Skillet

Ingredients:

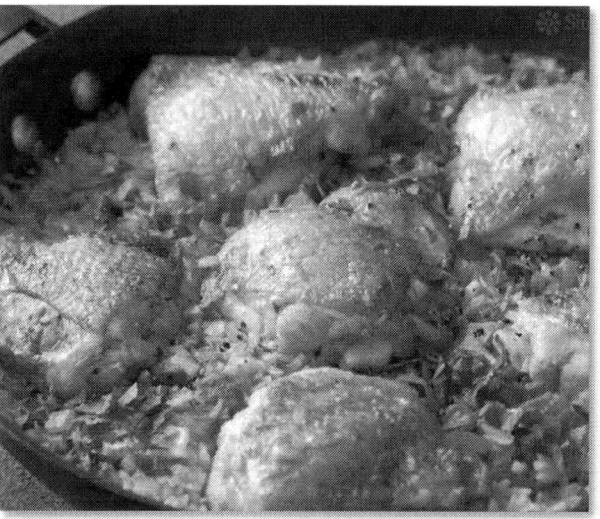

- ⅔ mug sliced leek, white and light green parts only
- 1 tablespoon herbs de Provence
- 3 mugs diced prepared chicken
- ¼ mug snipped fresh basil
- 2 tbsp snipped fresh mint
- 1 mug sliced off, seeded tomatoes
- ¼ mug Chicken Bone Broth
- ¼ mug dry white wine
- 1 0.5-ounce package dried chanterelle mushrooms
- 8 ounces fresh asparagus
- 2 tbsp olive oil
- 1 moderate bulb fennel, cored and thinly sliced
- 2 teaspoons finely shredded lemon peel
- 4 mugs roughly sliced off red or rainbow Swiss chard leaves

Instructions:

- Rehydrate dried mushrooms as per bundle Instructions, channel. Flush and channel once more; put in a safe spot. Then, snap off and eliminate woody bases from asparagus. Whenever wanted, scratch off scales. Predisposition cut asparagus into 2-inch pieces. In a huge sauce dish plan asparagus in bubbling water for 3 minutes or until fresh delicate; channel. Immediately dive into ice water to quit planning; put in a safe spot.
- In an extra-enormous skillet heat oil over moderate warmth. Supplement fennel, leek, and spices de Provence; get ready for 5 minutes or just until fennel starts to brown, shake ring sometimes. Supplement the rehydrated mushrooms, asparagus, chicken, tomatoes, Chicken Bone Broth, wine, and lemon strip. Bring to a stew.
- Wrap up and decrease warmth to low. Stew for 5 minutes or just until fennel and asparagus are delicate and tomatoes are succulent. Eliminate from heat. Shake in Swiss chard and let represent 2 minutes or until withered. Topping with basil and mint.

Smoky Portobello Mushrooms

Ingredients:

- ½ mug sliced off shallots
- 1 tablespoon chopped garlic
- 1-pound Swiss chard, stemmed and sliced off (about 10 mugs)
- 2 teaspoons Mediterranean Seasoning
- 4 large portobello mushrooms (about 1-pound total)
- ¼ mug olive oil

- 1 tablespoon Smoky Seasoning
- 2 tbsp olive oil
- ½ mug sliced off radishes

Instructions:

- Preheat stove to 400°F. Eliminate comes from mushrooms and save for Step 2. Utilize the tip of a spoon to scratch the gills out of the covers; eliminate gills. Put mushroom covers in a 3-quart rectangular heating dish; brush the two sides of mushrooms with the ¼ mug olive oil. Turn mushroom covers so the stemmed sides are up, Garnish with Smoky Seasoning. Wrap up preparing dish with foil. Heat, Wrap increased, around 20 minutes or until delicate. Then, slash held mushroom stems; put in a safe spot. To get ready chard, eliminate thick ribs from leaves and eliminate.
- Coarsely slash the chard leaves. In an extra-enormous skillet heat the 2 tbsp olive oil over moderate warmth. Addition shallots and garlic; get ready and shake for 30 seconds. Addition cut off mushroom stems, cut off chard, and Mediterranean Seasoning. Get ready, open up increased, for 6 to 8 minutes or until chard is delicate, shake ring once in a while. Appropriate chard joins among the mushroom covers. Sprinkle any fluid leftover in preparing dish overstuffed mushrooms. Top with cut off radishes.

Roasted Cabbage with Drizzle
Ingredients:

- ½ tsp. black pepper
- ⅓ mug balsamic vinegar
- 3 tbsp olive oil
- 1 small head cabbage, cored and slice into 8 wedges
- 2 teaspoons finely shredded orange peel

Instructions:

- Preheat oven to 450°F. Brush a large, rimmed baking sheet with 1 tablespoon of the olive oil. Organize cabbage wedges on the baking sheet. Brush cabbage with the remaining 2 tbsp olive oil and Garnish with pepper.
- Roast cabbage for 15 minutes. Turn cabbage wedges over; roast about 15 minutes more or until cabbage is tender and edges are golden brown. In a small sauce dish combine the balsamic vinegar and orange peel.

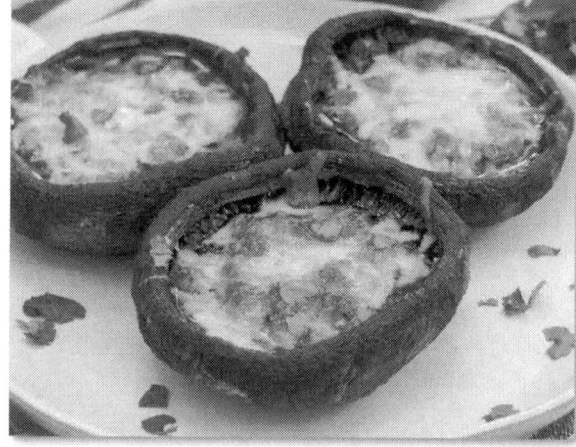

- Bring to boiling over moderate heat; reduce. Simmer, unwrap upped, about 4 minutes or until reduced by half. Drizzle over roasted cabbage wedges; serve instantly.

Mediterranean Radicchio

Ingredients:

- 1 tsp. Mediterranean Seasoning
- 2 large heads radicchio
- ¼ mug olive oil
- ¼ mug balsamic vinegar

Instructions:

- Preheat oven to 400°F. Quarter the radicchio, leaving some of the core attached (you should have 8 wedges). Brush slice sides of radicchio wedges with olive oil. Put wedges, slice sides down, on a baking sheet, Garnish with Mediterranean Seasoning.
- Roast about 15 minutes or until radicchio wilts, turning once halfway through roasting. Organize radicchio on a serving platter. Drizzle balsamic vinegar; serve instantly.

Roasted with Orange Vinaigrette

Ingredients:

- 2 tbsp white wine vinegar or champagne vinegar
- 2 tbsp apple cider
- 1 tsp. ground fennel seeds
- 1 tsp. finely shredded orange peel
- 6 tbsp extra virgin olive oil, plus more for brushing
- 1 large fennel bulb, trimmed, cored, and slice into wedges (reserve fronds for garnish if desired)
- 1 red onion, slice into wedges
- ½ of an orange, thinly sliced into rounds
- ½ mug orange juice
- ½ tsp. Dijon-Style Mustard
- Black pepper

Instructions:

- Preheat oven to 425°F. Brush a large baking sheet lightly with olive oil. Organize the fennel, onion, and orange slices on the baking sheet; drizzle with two tbsp of the olive oil. Gently fling vegetable to coat with oil. Roast vegetables for 25 to thirty minutes or till vegetables are tender and light golden, turning once halfway through roasting. Meanwhile, for orange vinaigrette, in a very blender combine orange juice, vinegar, apple cider, fennel seeds, orange peel, Dijon-Vogue Mustard, and pepper to style.
- With the blender running, slowly insert the remaining four tbsp olive oil in a very thin stream. Continue mixing until vinaigrette thickens. Shift vegetables to a serving platter. Drizzle vegetables with a number of the vinaigrette. If desired, garnish with reserved fennel fronds.

Cinnamon-Roasted Hindi Butternut

Ingredients:

- ¼ tsp. black pepper
- ⅛ tsp. cayenne pepper
- 1 butternut squash (about 2 pounds), peeled, seeded, and slice into ¾-inch cubes
- 2 tbsp olive oil
- ½ tsp. ground cinnamon

Instructions:

- Preheat oven to 400°F. In a large pot fling squash with olive oil, cinnamon, black pepper, and cayenne pepper. Line a large, rimmed baking sheet with parchment paper. Scatter squash in a single layer on the baking sheet. Roast for 30 to 35 minutes or until squash is tender and browned on edges, shake ring once or twice.

Broiled Asparagus and Pecans

Ingredients:

- 1 hard-prepared egg, peeled
- 3 tbsp sliced off pecans, toasted
- 1-pound fresh asparagus, trimmed
- 5 tbsp Roasted Garlic Vinaigrette
- Freshly ground black pepper

Instructions:

- Position oven rack 4 inches from heating part; preheat broiler to immense. Scatter asparagus spears on a baking sheet. Drizzle with 2 tbsp of the Roasted Garlic Vinaigrette. Using your hands, roll asparagus to coat with vinaigrette. Broil for 3 to five minutes or until blistered and tender, turning asparagus when every minute. Shift to a serving platter. Slice the egg in 0.5, press egg through a sieve over the asparagus.
- Drizzle asparagus and egg with the remaining three tbsp Roasted Garlic Vinaigrette. Top with pecans and Garnish with pepper.

Crunchy Cabbage Slaw and Mint

Ingredients:

- ¼ mug olive oil
- 4 mugs shredded cabbage
- 1½ mugs very thinly sliced radishes
- 1 mug cubed ripe mango
- 3 tbsp fresh lemon juice
- ¼ tsp. cayenne pepper
- ¼ tsp. ground cumin

- ½ mug bias-sliced scallions
- ⅓ mug sliced off fresh mint

Instructions:

- For dressing, in a large pot combine lemon juice, cayenne pepper, and ground cumin. Whisk in olive oil in a thin stream. Insert cabbage, radishes, mango, scallions, and mint to dressing in pot. Fling well to combine.

Roasted Cabbage Rounds and Lemon

Ingredients:

- 1 tsp. finely shredded lemon peel
- ¼ tsp. black pepper
- 1 tsp. caraway seeds
- 3 tbsp olive oil
- 1 moderate head cabbage, slice into 1-inch-thick rounds
- 2 teaspoons Dijon-Style Mustard
- Lemon wedges

Instructions:

- Preheat oven to 400°F. Brush a large, rimmed baking sheet with 1 tablespoon of the olive oil. Organize cabbage rounds on the baking sheet; set aside. In a tiny pot whisk along the remaining a pair of tbsp olive oil, Dijon-Style Mustard, and lemon peel.
- Brush over cabbage rounds on baking sheet, making certain mustard and lemon peel are evenly distributed. Garnish with pepper and caraway seeds. Roast for 30 to 35 minutes or until cabbage is tender and edges are golden brown. Serve with lemon wedges to press over cabbage.

Braised Cabbage and Toasted Walnuts

Ingredients:

- 1 mug Chicken Bone Broth
- ¾ mug Cashew Cream
- 4 teaspoons finely shredded lemon peel
- 4 teaspoons snipped fresh dill
- 3 tbsp olive oil
- 1 shallot, finely sliced off
- 1 small head green cabbage, slice into 6 wedges
- ½ tsp. black pepper
- 1 tablespoon finely sliced off scallions
- ¼ mug sliced off walnuts, toasted

Instructions:

- In an extra-huge skillet heat olive oil over moderate-huge warmth. Supplement shallot; plan for 2 to 3 minutes or until delicate and daintily caramelized. Addition cabbage wedges to skillet. Get ready, open up increased, for 10 minutes or until gently caramelized on each side, turning once partially through getting ready. Enhancement with pepper.
- Supplement Chicken Bone Broth to skillet. Bring to bubbling; diminish heat.
- Wrap up and stew for 25 to 30 minutes or until cabbage is delicate. In the interim, for Creamy Dill Sauce, in a little pot shake together Cashew Cream, lemon strip, dill, and scallions.
- To serve, move cabbage wedges to serving plates, shower with dish juices. Top with dill sauce and Garnish with toasted pecans.

Coarsely Roasted Cauliflower with Fennel

Ingredients:

- 1½ mugs frozen pearl onions, thawed and drained
- ¼ mug dried currants
- 2 teaspoons ground cumin
- 3 tbsp unrefined coconut oil
- 1 moderate head cauliflower, slice into florets (4 to 5 mugs)
- 2 heads fennel, coarsely sliced off
- Snipped fresh dill (optional)

Instructions:

- In an extra-large skillet heat coconut oil over moderate heat. Insert cauliflower, fennel, and pearl onions. Wrap up and prepare for 15 minutes, shake ring occasionally.
- Reduce heat to moderate-low. Insert currants and cumin to skillet; prepare, unwrap upped, about 10 minutes or until cauliflower and fennel are tender and golden brown. If desired, garnish with dill.

Indian-Style Savoy Cabbage

Ingredients:

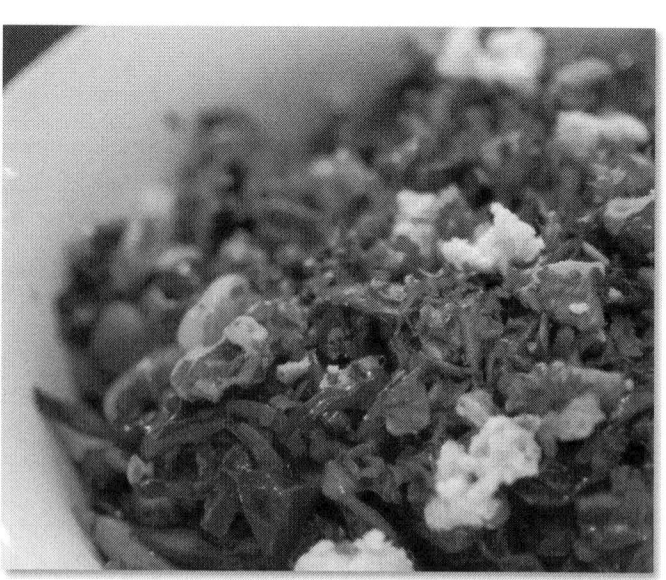

- 1 tsp. ground turmeric
- ½ mug Chicken Bone Broth
- 3 tbsp refined coconut oil
- 1 tablespoon black mustard seeds
- 1 3-inch cinnamon stick
- 2 mugs thinly sliced yellow onions (about 2 moderate)
- 12 mugs thinly sliced, cored savoy cabbage (about 1½ pounds)
- ½ mug snipped fresh cilantro (optional)
- 1 tsp. coriander seeds
- 1 2-inch knob fresh ginger, peeled and slice into ⅓-inch slices

- 5 cloves garlic
- 1 large jalapeño, stemmed, seeded, and halved
- 2 teaspoons notable salt-inserted garam masala
- 1 tsp. cumin seeds
- 1 whole bird's beak chile

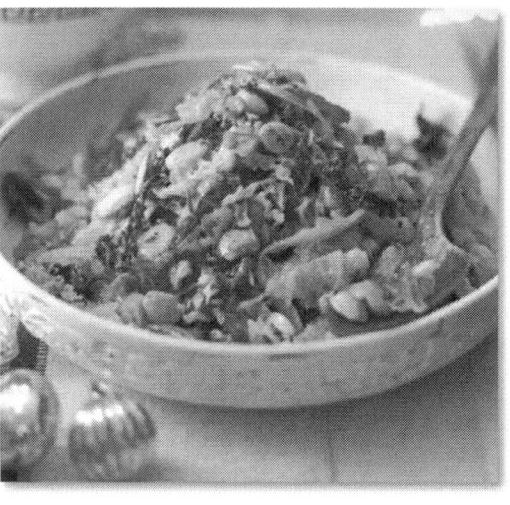

Instructions:

- In a food processor or blender combine ginger, garlic, jalapeño, garam masala, turmeric, and ¼ mug of the Chicken Bone Broth. Bring to a close and process or mix until sleek; set aside. In a further-giant skillet combine coconut oil, mustard seeds, coriander seeds, cumin seeds, chile, and cinnamon stick.
- Prepare over moderate-immense heat, shaking dish frequently, for two to three minutes or until the cinnamon stick unfurls. (Be careful-mustard seeds will pop and spatter as they prepare.) Insert onions; prepare and shake for five to six minutes or until onions are gently browned. Insert ginger combine.
- Prepare, for six to 8 minutes or until combine   is nicely caramelized, shake ring usually. Insert cabbage and therefore the remaining Chicken Bone Broth; combine well. Finish off and prepare concerning 15 minutes or till cabbage is tender, shake ring twice. Unwrap up skillet.
- Prepare and shake for 6 to seven minutes or till cabbage is gently browned and excess Chicken Bone Broth evaporates. Take away and remove cinnamon stick and chile. If desired, Garnish with cilantro.

Sautéed Green Toasted Sesame Seeds
Ingredients:

- 1 moderate tomato, sliced off
- 1 tablespoon chopped fresh ginger
- 3 cloves garlic, chopped
- ¼ tsp. crushed red pepper
- 2 tbsp sesame seeds
- 2 tbsp refined coconut oil
- 1 moderate onion, thinly sliced
- ½ of a 3- to 3½-pound head green cabbage, cored and very thinly sliced

Instructions:

- In an additional-large dry skillet toast sesame seeds over moderate heat for three to 4 minutes or till golden brown, shake ring almost constantly. Shift seeds to a small pot and funky fully. Shift seeds to a clean spice or occasional grinder; pulse to grind coarsely. Set ground sesame seeds aside.

- Meanwhile, in the same additional-large skillet heat coconut oil over moderate-immense heat. Insert onion; prepare regarding two minutes or simply till slightly soft. Shake in tomato, ginger, garlic, and crushed red pepper.
- Prepare and shake for two minutes a lot of. Insert sliced cabbage to tomato mix in skillet. Fling with tongs to mix. Prepare for twelve to 14 minutes or until cabbage is tender and just begins to brown, shake ring often. Insert ground sesame seeds; shake well to mix. Serve instantly.

Lemon Celery Soup with Herb Oil
Ingredients:

- ½ of a head cauliflower, cored and broken into florets
- ¼ mug packed Italian (flat leaf) parsley
- ¼ mug packed basil leaves
- ¼ mug olive oil
- 1 tablespoon fresh lemon juice
- 1 tablespoon olive oil
- 1 leek, sliced (white and light green parts only)
- 4 mugs Chicken Bone Broth
- ½ of a moderate celery root (about 10 ounces), peeled and slice into 1-inch cubes
- ¼ tsp. black pepper

Instructions:

- In an exceedingly large sauce dish heat the one tablespoon olive oil over moderate heat. Insert leek; prepare for four to 5 minutes or till tender. Insert Chicken Bone Broth, celery root, and cauliflower. Bring to boiling; reduce heat. Wrap up and simmer for 20 to twenty-five minutes or till vegetables are tender. Remove from heat; cool slightly.
- Meanwhile, for herb oil, in a food processor or blender combine the parsley, basil, and also the ¼ mug olive oil. Wrap up and method or blend till well combined and herbs are in very little items. Pour oil through a fine-mesh strainer into a small pot, pressing herbs with the back of a spoon to extract as abundant oil as possible.
- Remove herbs; set herb oil aside. Shift half of the celery root combine to the food processor or blender. Wrap up and process or blend till sleek. Pour into a large pot. Repeat with remaining celery root mix. Return all of the combine back to the sauce dish. Shake in lemon juice and pepper, heat through. Ladle soup into pots. Drizzle with herb oil.

Crunchy Chicken Wraps
Ingredients:

- 1 stalk celery
- 1 medium carrot
- 1/2 red bell pepper
- 1/4 cup low-fat mayonnaise
- 1/2 teaspoon onion powder
- 2 whole wheat lavash

- 8 ounces low-sodium canned chicken

Instructions:

- Dice celery, carrot and bell pepper.
- Combine the mayonnaise and onion powder in a small bowl.
- Spread 2 tablespoons of the mixture over each lavash flatbread.
- In a separate bowl combine the diced vegetables.
- Place half of the vegetables and 4 ounces of the chicken on one side of each flatbread.
- Roll up the flatbread and cut each one in half at a diagonal. Secure each half with a toothpick.
- Secure each tortilla half with a toothpick and cut each tortilla roll in half.

Shrimp Quesadilla
Ingredients:

- 5 ounces raw shrimp
- 2 tablespoons cilantro
- 1 tablespoon lemon juice
- 1/4 teaspoon ground cumin
- 1/8 teaspoon cayenne pepper
- 2 flour tortillas, burrito size
- 2 tablespoons sour cream
- 4 teaspoons salsa
- 2 tablespoons shredded jalapeno cheddar cheese

Instructions:

- Shell and devein shrimp. Rinse and cut into bite-size pieces. Chop cilantro.
- Combine cilantro, lemon juice, cumin and cayenne pepper in a zip-lock bag to make marinade. Add shrimp pieces and set aside to marinate for 5 minutes.
- Heat a skillet to medium heat and add shrimp with marinade. Stir-fry 1 to 2 minutes until shrimp turns orange. Remove skillet from heat and spoon shrimp out, leaving marinade.
- Add sour cream to marinade in skillet and stir to mix.
- Heat tortillas in a large skillet or microwave. Spread 2 teaspoons salsa onto each tortilla. Top with 1/2 shrimp mixture and sprinkle with 1 tablespoon cheese.
- Spoon 1 tablespoon sour cream marinade mixture on top of shrimp. Fold tortilla in half, turn over in skillet to heat, then remove from pan. Repeat with second tortilla and remaining shrimp, cheese and marinade.
- Cut each tortilla into 4 pieces. Garnish with cilantro and lemon wedge when ready to serve.

Soft Tacos with Mexican Seasoning
Ingredients:

- 1 recipe Mexican Seasoning
- 5 tablespoons onion
- 2 cups lettuce
- 1-pound ground beef
- 1/2 cup low-sodium tomato sauce
- 14 flour tortillas, 6-inch
- 5 tablespoons shredded sharp cheddar cheese

- 5 tablespoons sour cream

Instructions:

- Make the Mexican Seasoning recipe
- Chop the onion and lettuce.
- Brown and drain the ground beef. Add the seasoning mixture and the low-sodium tomato sauce. Heat over medium heat. Warm the tortillas.
- To assemble soft tacos, take 1 flour tortilla, add 1/4 cup seasoned ground beef, 1 teaspoon cheese, 1 teaspoon onion, 1 teaspoon sour cream and lettuce as desired.

Tortilla Beef Rollups (High Protein)
Ingredients:

- 2 flour tortilla, 6" size
- 2 tablespoons whipped cream cheese
- 5 ounces roast beef, cooked
- 1/4 cup red onion, chopped
- 1/4 sweet bell pepper (red, yellow or green), cut in strips
- 8 cucumber slices

Instructions:

- Spread cream cheese over tortillas.
- Divide ingredients in half to make two tortillas. Layer each tortilla with roast beef, red onion, pepper strips, cucumbers and lettuce.
- Roll up like a jellyroll.
- Slice each tortilla into 4 pieces or serve whole. Romaine lettuce leaves

Turkey Waldorf Salad
Ingredients:

- 12 ounces unsalted turkey breast, cooked
- 3 medium red apples
- 1 cup celery
- 1/2 cup onion
- 1/4 cup mayonnaise
- 2 tablespoons apple juice

Instructions:

- Cut turkey into cubes. Dice celery and apples; finely chop onion.
- In a medium bowl, combine turkey, apple, celery and onion.
- Add mayonnaise and apple juice. Stir together until well mixed.
- Chill until ready to serve.

Leaf Lettuce and Carrot Salad with Basilic Vinaigrette
Ingredients:

FOR THE VINAIGRETTE

- ½ cup olive oil

- 4 tablespoons balsamic vinegar
- 2 tablespoons chopped fresh oregano
- Pinch red pepper flakes
- Freshly ground black pepper

FOR THE SALAD

- 4 cups shredded green leaf lettuce
- 1 carrot, shredded
- ¾ cup fresh green beans, cut into 1-inch pieces
- 3 large radishes, sliced thin

Instructions:

TO MAKE THE VINAIGRETTE

- In a small bowl, whisk together the olive oil, balsamic vinegar, oregano,
- and red pepper flakes.
- Season with pepper.

TO MAKE THE SALAD

- In a large bowl, toss together the lettuce, carrot, green beans, and radishes.
- Add the vinaigrette to the vegetables and toss to coat.
- Arrange the salad on 4 plates to serve.

Strawberry Watercress Salad with Almond Dressing

Ingredients:

FOR THE DRESSING

- ¼ cup olive oil
- ¼ cup rice vinegar
- 1 tablespoon honey
- ¼ teaspoon pure almond extract
- ¼ teaspoon ground mustard
- Freshly ground black pepper

FOR THE SALAD

- 2 cups roughly chopped watercress
- 2 cups shredded green leaf lettuce
- ½ red onion, sliced very thin
- ½ English cucumber, chopped
- 1 cup sliced strawberries

Instructions:

TO MAKE THE DRESSING

- In a small bowl, whisk together the olive oil and rice vinegar until
- emulsified.
- Whisk in the honey, almond extract, mustard, and pepper; set aside.

TO MAKE THE SALAD

- In a large bowl, toss together the watercress, green leaf lettuce, onion, cucumber, and strawberries.
- Pour the dressing over the salad and toss to combine.

LEMON DRESSING

Ingredients:

- ¼ cup heavy cream
- ¼ cup freshly squeezed lemon juice
- 2 tablespoons granulated sugar
- 2 tablespoons chopped fresh dill
- 2 tablespoons finely chopped scallion, green part only
- ¼ teaspoon freshly ground black pepper
- 1 English cucumber, sliced thin
- 2 cups shredded green cabbage

Instructions:

- In a small bowl, stir together the cream, lemon juice, sugar, dill, scallion,
- and pepper until well blended.
- In a large bowl, toss together the cucumber and cabbage.
- Place the salad in the refrigerator and chill for 1 hour.
- Stir before serving.

Leaf Lettuce and Asparagus Salad with Raspberries

Ingredients:

- 2 cups shredded green leaf lettuce
- 1 cup asparagus, cut into long ribbons with a peeler
- 1 scallion, both green and white parts, sliced
- 1 cup raspberries
- 2 tablespoons balsamic vinegar
- Freshly ground black pepper

Instructions:

- Arrange the lettuce evenly on 4 serving plates.
- Arrange the asparagus and scallion on top of the greens.
- Place the raspberries on top of the salads, dividing the berries evenly.
- Drizzle the salads with balsamic vinegar.
- Season with pepper.

Waldorg Salad

Ingredients:

- 3 cups green leaf lettuce, torn into pieces
- 1 cup halved grapes
- 3 celery stalks, chopped
- 1 large apple, cored, peeled, and chopped

- ½ cup light sour cream
- 2 tablespoons freshly squeezed lemon juice
- 1 tablespoon granulated sugar

Instructions:

- Arrange the lettuce evenly on 4 plates; set aside.
- In a small bowl, stir together the grapes, celery, and apple.
- In another small bowl, stir together the sour cream, lemon juice, and sugar.
- Add the sour cream mixture to the grape mixture and stir to coat.
- Spoon the dressed grape mixture onto each plate, dividing the mixture
- evenly.

Asian Pear Salad

Ingredients:

- 2 cups finely shredded green cabbage
- 1 cup finely shredded red cabbage
- 2 scallions, both green and white parts, chopped
- 2 celery stalks, chopped
- 1 Asian pear, cored and grated
- ½ red bell pepper, boiled and chopped
- ½ cup chopped cilantro
- ¼ cup olive oil
- Juice of 1 lime
- Zest of 1 lime
- 1 teaspoon granulated sugar

Instructions:

- In a large bowl, toss together the green and red cabbage, scallions, celery,
- pear, red pepper, and cilantro.
- In a small bowl, whisk together the olive oil, lime juice, lime zest, and
- sugar.
- Add the dressing to the cabbage mixture and toss to combine.
- Chill for 1 hour in the refrigerator before serving.

Couscous Salad with Spicy Citrus Dressing

Ingredients:

- FOR THE DRESSING
- ¼ cup olive oil
- 3 tablespoons freshly squeezed grapefruit juice
- Juice of 1 lime
- Zest of 1 lime
- 1 tablespoon chopped fresh parsley
- Pinch cayenne pepper
- Freshly ground black pepper

FOR THE SALAD

- 3 cups cooked couscous, chilled
- ½ red bell pepper, chopped
- 1 scallion, both white and green parts, chopped
- 1 apple, cored and chopped

Instructions:

TO MAKE THE DRESSING

- In a small bowl, whisk together the olive oil, grapefruit juice, lime juice,
- lime zest, parsley, and cayenne pepper.
- Season with black pepper.

TO MAKE THE SALAD

- In a large bowl, mix together the chilled couscous, red pepper, scallion, and
- apple.
- Add the dressing to the couscous mixture and toss to combine.
- Chill in the refrigerator for at least 1 hour before serving.

Tabbouleh
Ingredients:

- 4 cups cooked white rice
- ½ red bell pepper, boiled and finely chopped
- ½ yellow bell pepper, boiled and chopped
- ½ zucchini, finely chopped, boiled until tender
- 1 cup chopped eggplant, boiled until tender
- ¼ cup finely chopped fresh parsley
- ¼ cup finely chopped fresh cilantro
- 2 tablespoons olive oil
- Juice of 1 lemon
- Zest of 1 lemon
- Freshly ground black pepper

Instructions:

- In a large bowl, stir together the rice, red bell pepper, yellow bell pepper, zucchini, eggplant, parsley, cilantro, olive oil, lemon juice, and lemon zest until well combined.
- Season with pepper.
- Chill the salad in the refrigerator for at least 1 hour before serving.

Ginger Beef Salad
Ingredients:

FOR THE BEEF

- 2 tablespoons olive oil
- 2 tablespoons freshly squeezed lime juice
- 1 tablespoon grated fresh ginger
- 2 teaspoons minced garlic
- ½ pound flank steak

- FOR THE VINAIGRETTE
- ¼ cup olive oil
- ¼ cup rice vinegar
- Juice of 1 lime
- Zest of 1 lime
- 1 tablespoon honey
- 1 teaspoon chopped fresh thyme

FOR THE SALAD

- 4 cups torn green leaf lettuce
- ½ red onion, sliced thin
- ½ cup sliced radishes

Instructions:

TO MAKE THE BEEF

- In a small bowl, stir together the olive oil, lime juice, ginger, and garlic until well blended.
- Add the flank steak to the marinade and turn it to coat both sides of the meat.
- Cover the bowl with plastic wrap and place in the refrigerator for 1 hour to marinate.
- Remove the steak from the marinade and discard the marinade.
- Preheat a barbecue to medium-high and grill the steak to medium doneness, turning once, for about 5 minutes per side, depending on the thickness of the steak.
- Remove the steak; place on a cutting board and let the meat rest for 10 minutes.
- Slicing the meat thinly across the grain.

TO MAKE THE VINAIGRETTE

- In a small bowl, whisk together the olive oil, rice vinegar, lime juice, lime zest,
- honey, and thyme; set aside.

TO MAKE THE SALAD

- Arrange the lettuce, onion, and radishes on 6 plates, dividing evenly.
- Drizzle each salad with vinaigrette.
- Top each salad with the sliced beef.

Red Pepper Strata

Ingredients:

- Butter, for greasing the baking dish
- 8 slices fresh white bread, cut into cubes
- 1 tablespoon unsalted butter
- ½ sweet onion, chopped
- 1 teaspoon minced garlic
- 1 red bell pepper, boiled and chopped
- 6 eggs
- ¼ cup tarragon vinegar
- 1 cup rice milk
- 1 teaspoon Tabasco sauce
- ½ teaspoon freshly ground black pepper
- 1-ounce Parmesan cheese, grated

Instructions:

- Preheat the oven to 250°F.
- Lightly grease a 9-by-9-inch baking dish with butter; set aside.
- Line a baking sheet with parchment paper and scatter the bread cubes on the sheet.
- Bake the bread cubes for about 10 minutes or until they are crisp.
- Remove the bread cubes from the oven; set aside.
- In a medium skillet over medium-high heat, melt the butter.
- Sauté the onion and garlic for about 3 minutes or until softened.
- Add the red pepper and sauté an additional 2 minutes.
- Spread half of the bread cubes in a layer in the baking dish and top with half of the sautéed vegetables.
- Repeat with the remaining half of the bread cubes and vegetables.
- In a medium bowl, whisk together the eggs, vinegar, rice milk, hot sauce, and pepper.
- Pour the egg mixture evenly into the baking dish.
- Cover the dish and place in the fridge to soak for at least 2 hours or overnight.
- Let the strata come to room temperature.
- Preheat the oven to 325°F.
- Remove the plastic wrap and bake for about 45 minutes or until golden.
- Sprinkle the top of the strata with cheese and bake an additional 5 minutes.
- Serve hot.

Couscous Burger

Ingredients:

- ½ cup canned chickpeas, rinsed and drained
- 2 tablespoons chopped fresh cilantro
- 2 tablespoons chopped fresh parsley
- 1 tablespoon freshly squeezed lemon juice
- 2 teaspoons lemon zest
- 1 teaspoon minced garlic
- 2½ cups cooked couscous
- 2 eggs, lightly beaten
- 2 tablespoons olive oil

Instructions:

- Put the chickpeas, cilantro, parsley, lemon juice, lemon zest, and garlic in a food processor and pulse until a paste forms (or use a large bowl and a handheld immersion blender).
- Transfer the chickpea mixture to a bowl and add the couscous and eggs, mixing thoroughly to combine.
- Chill the mixture in the refrigerator for 1 hour to firm it. Form the couscous mixture into 4 patties.
- Place a large skillet over medium-high heat and add the olive oil.
- Place the patties in the skillet, 2 at a time, gently pressing them down with
- the back of a spatula. Cook for 5 minutes or until golden and flip the patties over.
- Cook the other side for 5 minutes and transfer the cooked burgers to a plate covered with a paper towel.
- Repeat with the remaining 2 burgers.

Marinated Tofu Stir-fry

Ingredients:

FOR THE TOFU

- 1 tablespoon freshly squeezed lemon juice
- 1 teaspoon minced garlic
- 1 teaspoon grated fresh ginger
- Pinch red pepper flakes
- 5 ounces extra-firm tofu, pressed well and cubed (see ingredient tip)

FOR THE STIR-FRY

- 1 tablespoon olive oil
- ½ cup cauliflower florets
- ½ cup thinly sliced carrots
- ½ cup julienned red pepper
- ½ cup fresh green beans
- 2 cups cooked white rice

Instructions:

TO MAKE THE TOFU

- In a small bowl, mix together the lemon juice, garlic, ginger, and red pepper
- flakes.
- Add the tofu and toss to coat.
- Place the bowl in the refrigerator and marinate for 2 hours.

TO MAKE THE STIR FRY

- In a large skillet over medium-high heat, heat the oil.
- Sauté the tofu for about 8 minutes or until it is lightly browned and heated
- through.
- Add the cauliflower and carrots and sauté for 5 minutes, stirring and tossing constantly.
- Add the red pepper and green beans; sauté for 3 additional minutes.
- Serve over the white rice.

Thai inspired Vegetable Curry

Ingredients:

- 2 teaspoons olive oil
- ½ sweet onion, diced
- 2 teaspoons minced garlic
- 2 teaspoons grated fresh ginger
- ½ eggplant, peeled and diced
- 1 carrot, peeled and diced
- 1 red bell pepper, diced
- 1 tablespoon Hot Curry Powder (here)
- 1 teaspoon ground cumin

- ½ teaspoon coriander
- Pinch cayenne pepper
- 1½ cups homemade vegetable stock
- 1 tablespoon cornstarch
- ¼ cup water

Instructions:

- In a large stockpot over medium-high heat, heat the oil.
- Sauté the onion, garlic, and ginger for 3 minutes or until they are softened.
- Add the eggplant, carrots, and red pepper, and sauté, stirring often, for 6 additional minutes.
- Stir in the curry powder, cumin, coriander, cayenne pepper, and vegetable stock.
- Bring the curry to a boil and then reduce the heat to low.
- Simmer the curry for about 30 minutes or until the vegetables are tender.
- In a small bowl, stir together the cornstarch and water.
- Stir the cornstarch mixture into the curry and simmer for about 5 minutes or until the sauce is thickened.

Tofu and Eggplant Stir-Fry

Ingredients:

- 1 tablespoon granulated sugar
- 1 tablespoon all-purpose flour
- 1 teaspoon grated fresh ginger
- 1 teaspoon minced garlic
- 1 teaspoon minced jalapeño pepper
- Juice of 1 lime
- Water
- 2 tablespoons olive oil, divided
- 5 ounces extra-firm tofu, cut into ½-inch cubes
- 2 cups cubed eggplant
- 2 scallions, both green and white parts, sliced
- 3 tablespoons chopped cilantro

Instructions:

- In a small bowl, whisk together the sugar, flour, ginger, garlic, jalapeño,
- lime juice, and enough water to make ⅔ cup of sauce; set aside.
- In a large skillet over medium-high heat, heat 1 tablespoon of the oil.
- Sauté the tofu for about 6 minutes or until it is crisp and golden.
- Remove the tofu; set aside on a plate.
- Add the remaining 1 tablespoon oil and sauté the eggplant cubes for about 10 minutes or until they are fully cooked and lightly browned.
- Add the tofu and scallions to the skillet and toss to combine.
- Pour in the sauce and bring to a boil, stirring constantly, for about 2 minutes or until the sauce is thickened.
- Add the cilantro before serving.

Mie Goreng with Broccoli

Ingredients:

- ½ pound rice noodles
- ¼ cup packed dark brown sugar
- 2 teaspoons minced garlic
- 1 teaspoon grated fresh ginger
- 1 teaspoon low-sodium soy sauce
- ½ teaspoon sambal Oelek
- 4 ounces extra-firm tofu, cut into ½-inch cubes
- 1 tablespoon cornstarch
- 2 tablespoons olive oil, divided
- 2 cups broccoli, cut into small florets
- 2 scallions, both green and white parts, sliced thin on the diagonal
- Lime wedges, for garnish

Instructions:

- Cook the noodles according to the package instructions; drain and set aside.
- In a small bowl, whisk together the brown sugar, garlic, ginger, soy sauce, and sambal Oelek; set aside.
- Drain the tofu on paper towels for 30 minutes and pat the tofu dry.
- Toss the tofu with the cornstarch and shake to remove the excess.
- In a large skillet over medium-high heat, heat 1 tablespoon of the olive oil.
- Add the tofu and sauté for about 10 minutes or until the tofu is browned on all sides and crispy.
- Transfer the tofu to a plate with a slotted spoon.
- Add the remaining 1 tablespoon oil to the skillet.
- Sauté the broccoli for about 4 minutes or until it is tender.
- Add the sauce and tofu to the skillet and cook for about 2 minutes or until
- the sauce thickens.
- Serve topped with scallions and garnish with lime wedges.

Grilled Shrimp with Cucumber Lime Salsa

Ingredients:

- 2 tablespoons olive oil
- 6 ounces large shrimp (16 to 20 count), peeled and deveined, tails left on
- 1 teaspoon minced garlic
- ½ cup chopped English cucumber
- ½ cup chopped mango
- Zest of 1 lime
- Juice of 1 lime
- Freshly ground black pepper
- Lime wedges for garnish
- Soak 4 wooden skewers in water for 30 minutes.

Instructions:

- Preheat the barbecue to medium-high heat.
- In a large bowl, toss together the olive oil, shrimp, and garlic.

- Thread the shrimp onto the skewers, about 4 shrimp per skewer.
- In a small bowl, stir together the cucumber, mango, lime zest, and lime juice, and season the salsa lightly with pepper. Set aside.
- Grill the shrimp for about 10 minutes, turning once or until the shrimp is opaque and cooked through.
- Season the shrimp lightly with pepper.
- Serve the shrimp on the cucumber salsa with lime wedges on the side.

Crab Cake with Lime Salsa

Ingredients:

FOR THE SALSA

- ½ English cucumber, diced
- 1 lime, chopped
- ½ cup boiled and chopped red bell pepper
- 1 teaspoon chopped fresh cilantro
- Freshly ground black pepper

FOR THE CRAB CAKES

- 8 ounces queen crab meat
- ¼ cup breadcrumbs
- 1 small egg
- ¼ cup boiled and chopped red bell pepper
- 1 scallion, both green and white parts, minced
- 1 tablespoon chopped fresh parsley
- Splash hot sauce
- Olive oil spray, for the pan

Instructions:

TO MAKE THE SALSA

- In a small bowl, stir together the cucumber, lime, red pepper, and cilantro.
- Season with pepper; set aside.
- TO MAKE THE CRAB CAKES
- In a medium bowl, mix together the crab, breadcrumbs, egg, red pepper, scallion, parsley, and hot sauce until it holds together. Add more breadcrumbs, if necessary.
- Form the crab mixture into 4 patties and place them on a plate.
- Refrigerate the crab cakes for 1 hour to firm them.
- Spray a large skillet generously with olive oil spray and place it over medium-high heat.
- Cook the crab cakes in batches, turning, for about 5 minutes per side or until golden brown.
- Serve the crab cakes with the salsa.

Seafood Casserole

Ingredients:

- 2 cups eggplant, peeled and diced into 1-inch pieces
- Butter, for greasing the baking dish
- 1 tablespoon olive oil
- ½ small, sweet onion, chopped

- 1 teaspoon minced garlic
- 1 celery stalk, chopped
- ½ red bell pepper, boiled and chopped
- 3 tablespoons freshly squeezed lemon juice
- 1 teaspoon hot sauce
- ¼ teaspoon Creole Seasoning Mix (here)
- ½ cup white rice, uncooked
- 1 large egg
- 4 ounces cooked shrimp

Instructions:

- Preheat the oven to 350°F.
- In a small saucepan filled with water over medium-high heat, boil the
- eggplant for 5 minutes. Drain and set aside in a large bowl.
- Grease a 9-by-13-inch baking dish with butter and set aside.
- In a large skillet over medium heat, heat the olive oil.
- Sauté the onion, garlic, celery, and bell pepper for about 4 minutes or until
- they are tender.
- Add the sautéed vegetables to the eggplant, along with the lemon juice, hot
- sauce, Creole seasoning, rice, and egg. ounces queen crab meat
- Stir to combine.
- Fold in the shrimp and crab meat.
- Spoon the casserole mixture into the casserole dish, patting down the top.
- Bake for 25 to 30 minutes or until the casserole is heated through and the
- rice is tender.
- Serve warm.

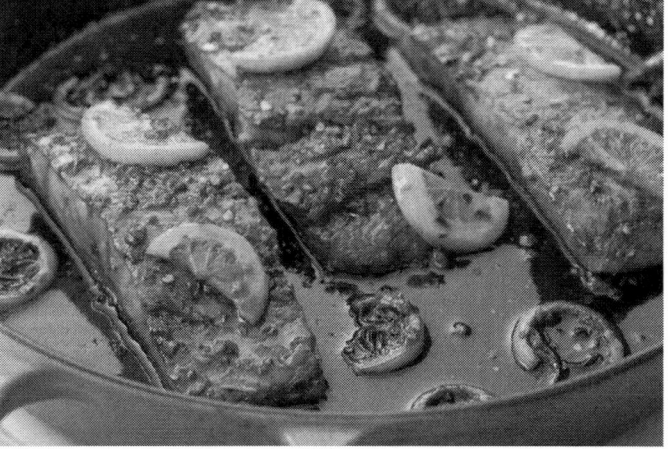

Sweet Glazed Salmon

Ingredients:

- 2 tablespoons honey
- 1 teaspoon lemon zest
- ½ teaspoon freshly ground black pepper
- 4 (3-ounce) salmon fillets
- 1 tablespoon olive oil
- ½ scallion, white and green parts, chopped

Instructions:

- In a small bowl, stir together the honey, lemon zest, and pepper.
- Wash the salmon and pat dry with paper towels.
- Rub the honey mixture all over each fillet.
- In a large skillet over medium heat, heat the olive oil.
- Add the salmon fillets and cook the salmon for about 10 minutes, turning once, or until it is lightly browned and just cooked through.
- Serve topped with chopped scallion.

Chapter 4: Dinner Recipes

Fish Pie
Ingredients:

- 3 interlock fillets and slice into moderate pieces
- 2 bay leaves
- ¼ mug ghee+ 2 tbsp ghee
- A pinch of nutmeg, ground
- 1 tsp. Dijon mustard
- 1 mug cheddar cheese, shredded+ ½ mug cheddar cheese, shredded
- 1 cauliflower head, florets separated
- 4 eggs
- 1 red onion, sliced off
- 2 salmon fillets, skinless and slice into moderate pieces
- 2 mackerel fillets, skinless and slice into moderate pieces
- 4 cloves
- 1 mug whipping cream
- ½ mug water
- Some sliced off parsley

- Table salt and black pepper to the taste
- 4 tbsp chives, sliced off

Instructions:

- Put some water in an exceedingly dish, insert some table salt, bring to a boil over moderate heat, insert eggs, prepare them for 10 minutes, take away heat, drain, leave them to chill down, peel and slice them into quarters.
- Put water in another pot, bring to a boil, insert cauliflower florets, prepare for 10 minutes, drain them, shift to your blender, insert ¼ mug ghee, pulse well and shift to a pot.
- Put cream and ½ mug water in an exceedingly dish, insert fish, fling to coat and Warm up over moderate heat. Insert onion, cloves and bay leaves, bring to a boil, scale back heat and simmer for 10 minutes. Remove heat, shift fish to a baking dish and leave aside. come dish with fish sauce to heat, insert nutmeg, shake and prepare for 5 minutes.
- Take away heat, remove cloves and bay leaves, insert one mug cheddar cheese and a couple of tbsp ghee and shake well.
- Put egg quarters on prime of the fish within the baking dish. Insert cream and cheese sauce over them, prime with cauliflower mash, Garnish the rest of the cheddar cheese, chives and parsley, introduce in the oven at 400 degrees F for 30 minutes. Leave the pie to cool down twenty-five a touch before slicing and serving.

Baked Fish
Ingredients:

- Table salt and black pepper to the taste
- 2 tbsp mayonnaise
- 1 tsp. dill weed
- Preparing spray
- 1-pound interlock
- 3 teaspoons water
- 2 tbsp lemon juice
- A pinch of old bay seasoning

Instructions:

- Spray a baking dish with some preparing oil. Insert lemon juice, water and fish and fling to coat a bit. Insert table salt, pepper, old bay seasoning, and dill weed and fling again. Insert mayo and Scatter well.
- Introduce in the oven at 350 degrees F and bake for 30 minutes. Distribute between plates and serve.

Green Tilapia
Ingredients:

- 4 tbsp mayonnaise

- ¼ tsp. basil, dried
- ¼ tsp. garlic grinding grains
- 2 tbsp lemon juice
- 4 tilapia fillets, boneless
- Table salt and black pepper to the taste
- ½ mug parmesan, grated
- 4 tilapia fillets, boneless
- Table salt and black pepper to the taste
- ½ mug parmesan, grated
- ¼ mug ghee
- Preparing spray
- A pinch of onion grinding grains

Instructions:

- Spray a baking sheet with preparing spray, put tilapia on it, season with table salt and pepper, introduce in preheated broiler and prepare for 3 minutes. Turn fish on the other side and broil for 3 minutes more.
- In a pot, combine parmesan with mayo, basil, garlic, lemon juice, onion grinding grains and ghee and shake well. Insert fish to this combine, fling to coat well, Put on baking sheet again and broil for 3 minutes more. Shift to plates and serve.

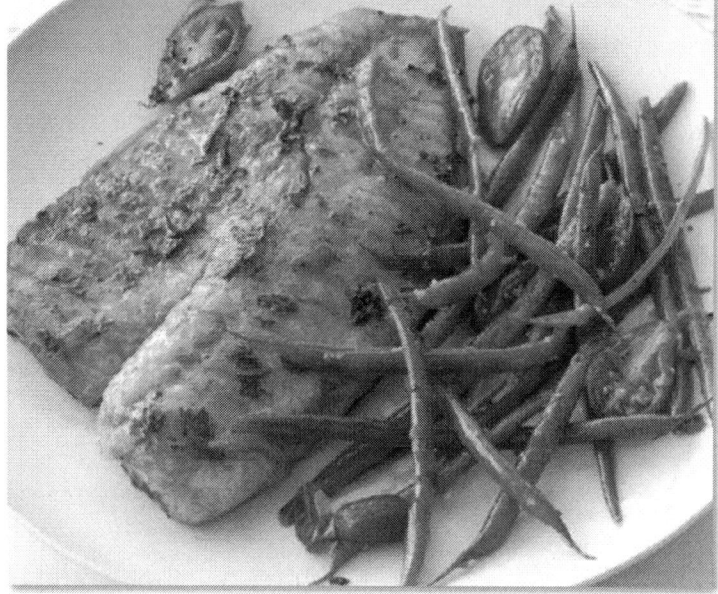

Amazing Trout and Special Sauce
Ingredients:

- 1 tablespoon ghee
- Zest and juice from 1 orange
- A handful parsley, sliced off
- 1 big trout fillet
- Table salt and black pepper to the taste
- 1 tablespoon olive oil
- ½ mug pecans, sliced off

Instructions:

- Warm up a dish with the oil over moderate immense heat, insert the fish fillet, season with table salt and pepper, prepare for 4 minutes on each side, shift to a plate and keep warm for now. Warm up the same dish with the ghee over moderate heat, insert pecans, shake and toast for 1 minutes.

- Insert orange juice and zest, some table salt and pepper and sliced off parsley, shake, prepare for 1 minute and pour over fish fillet. Serve right away.

Salmon Fish with Caper Sauce

Ingredients:

- 1 tablespoon Italian seasoning
- 2 tbsp capers
- 3 tbsp lemon juice
- 4 garlic cloves, chopped
- 3 salmon fillets
- Table salt and black pepper to the taste
- 1 tablespoon olive oil
- 2 tbsp ghee

Instructions:

- Warm up a dish with the olive oil over moderate heat, insert fish fillets skin side up, season them with table salt, pepper and Italian seasoning, prepare for 2 minutes, flip and prepare for 2 additional minutes, take away heat, finish off dish and leave aside for 15 minutes. Shift fish to a plate and leave them aside.
- Warm up the same dish over moderate heat, insert capers, lemon juice and garlic, shake and prepare for two minutes. Take the dish off the warmth, insert ghee and shake terribly well. Return fish to dish and fling to coat with the sauce. Distribute between plates and serve.

Grilled Oysters

Ingredients:

- 1 tablespoon parsley
- A pinch of sweet paprika
- 6 big oysters, shucked
- 3 garlic cloves, chopped
- 1 lemon slice in wedges
- 2 tbsp melted ghee

Instructions:

- Top each oyster with melted ghee, parsley, paprika and ghee. Put them on preheated grill over moderate immense heat and prepare for 8 minutes. Serve them with lemon wedges on the side.

Delicious Trout and Ghee Sauce

Ingredients:

- 3 tbsp chives, sliced off
- 6 tbsp ghee

- 2 tbsp olive oil
- 4 trout fillets
- Table salt and black pepper to the taste
- 3 teaspoons lemon zest, grated
- 2 teaspoons lemon juice

Instructions:

- Season trout with table salt and pepper, drizzle the olive oil and massage a bit. Warm up your kitchen grill over moderate immense heat, insert fish fillets, prepare for 4 minutes, flip and prepare for 4 minutes more.
- Meanwhile, Warm up a dish with the ghee over moderate heat, insert table salt, pepper, chives, lemon juice and zest and shake well. Distribute fish fillets on plates, drizzle the ghee sauce over them and serve.

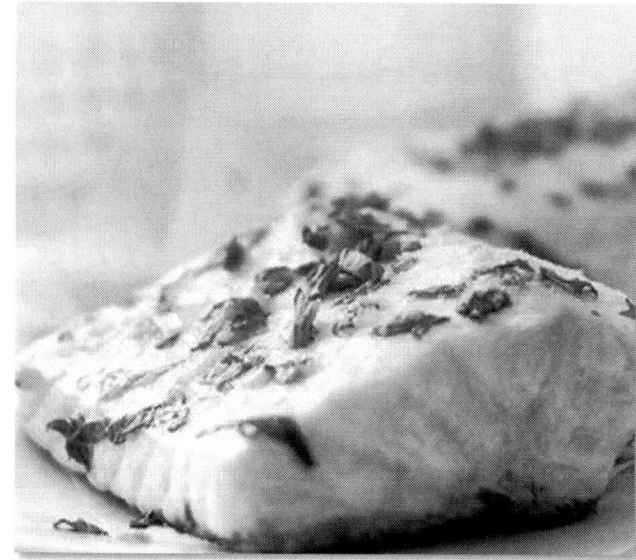

Mayonnaise Baked Halibut
Ingredients:

- 2 tbsp green onions, sliced off
- 6 garlic cloves, chopped
- A dash of Tabasco sauce
- 4 halibut fillets
- ½ mug parmesan, grated
- ¼ mug ghee
- ¼ mug mayonnaise
- Table salt and black pepper to the taste
- Juice of ½ lemon

Instructions:

- Season halibut with table salt, pepper and some of the lemon juice, place in a very baking dish and prepare in the oven at 450 degrees F for 6 minutes. Meanwhile, Warm up a dish with the ghee over moderate heat, insert parmesan, mayo, inexperienced onions, Tabasco sauce, garlic and the rest of the lemon juice and shake well.
- Take fish out of the oven, drizzle parmesan sauce all over, flip oven to broil and broil your fish for three minutes. Distribute between plates and serve.

Asian Green Sauce Salmon
Ingredients:

- 2 ounces Kimchi, finely sliced off
- Table salt and black pepper to the taste

- 2 tbsp ghee, soft
- 1 and ¼ pound salmon fillet

Instructions:

- In your food processor, combine ghee with Kimchi and blend well. Rub salmon with table salt, pepper and Kimchi combine and Put into a baking dish.
- Introduce in the oven at 425 degrees F and bake for 15 minutes. Distribute between plates and serve with a side salad.

Crusted Salmon Fillet
Ingredients:

- Table salt and black pepper to the taste
- ½ mug parmesan, grated
- 3 garlic cloves, chopped
- 2 pounds salmon
- ¼ mug parsley, sliced off

Instructions:

- Put salmon on a lined baking sheet, season with table salt and pepper, wrap up with a parchment paper, introduce in the oven at 425 degrees F and bake for 10 minutes.
- Take fish out of the oven, Garnish parmesan, parsley and garlic over fish, introduce in the oven again and prepare for 5 minutes more. Distribute between plates and serve.

Grilled Salmon Limes
Ingredients:

- 1 tsp. sweet paprika
- ½ tsp. ancho chili grinding grains
- 1 tsp. onion grinding grains
- 2 tbsp cilantro, sliced off
- Juice from 2 limes
- Table salt and black pepper to the taste
- 1 small red onion, sliced off
- 4 salmon fillets
- 1 tablespoon olive oil
- Table salt and black pepper to the taste
- 1 tsp. cumin, ground
- 1 avocado, pitted, peeled and sliced off

Instructions:

- In a pot, combine table salt, pepper, chili grinding grains, onion grinding grains, paprika and cumin. Rub salmon with this combine, drizzle the oil and rub again and prepare on preheated grill for 4 minutes on each side.

- Meanwhile, in a pot, combine avocado with red onion, table salt, pepper, cilantro and lime juice and shake. Distribute salmon between plates and top each fillet with avocado salsa.

Tuna Cakes Parsley

Ingredients:

- ½ mug red onion, sliced off
- 1 tsp. garlic grinding grains
- Table salt and black pepper to the taste
- 15 ounces canned tuna, drain well and flaked
- 3 eggs
- ½ tsp. dill, dried
- 1 tsp. parsley, dried
- Oil for frying

Instructions:

- In a pot, combine tuna with table salt, pepper, dill, parsley, onion, garlic grinding grains and eggs and shake well. Shape your cakes and Put on a plate.
- Warm up a dish with some oil over moderate immense heat, insert tuna cakes, prepare for 5 minutes on each side. Distribute between plates and serve.

Cod Balsamic Vinegar

Ingredients:

- 3 garlic cloves, chopped
- 3 tbsp soy sauce
- 1 mug fish stock
- 1-pound cod, slice into moderate pieces
- Table salt and black pepper to the taste
- 2 green onions, sliced off
- 1 tablespoon balsamic vinegar
- 1 tablespoon ginger, grated
- ½ tsp. chili pepper, crushed

Instructions:

- Warm up a dish over moderate immense heat, insert fish pieces and brown it a few minutes on each side. Insert garlic, green onions, table salt, pepper, soy sauce, fish stock, vinegar, chili pepper and ginger, shake, wrap up, reduce heat and prepare for 20 minutes. Distribute between plates and serve.

Tasty Sea Bass Fillet with Capers

Ingredients:

- 2 tbsp capers
- 2 tbsp dill
- 1 lemon, sliced
- 1-pound sea bass fillet
- Table salt and black pepper to the taste

Instructions:

- Put sea bass fillet into a baking dish, season with table salt and pepper, insert capers, dill and lemon slices on top. Introduce in the oven at 350 degrees F and bake for 15 minutes. Distribute between plates and serve.

Delicious Salmon Meatballs

Ingredients:

- 1 egg
- 2 tbsp Dijon mustard
- 1 tablespoon coconut flour
- Table salt and black pepper to the taste
- For the sauce:
- 4 garlic cloves, chopped
- Juice and zest of 1 lemon
- 2 mugs coconut cream
- 2 tbsp chives, sliced off
- 2 tbsp ghee
- 2 garlic cloves, chopped
- 1/3 mug onion, sliced off
- 1-pound wild salmon, boneless and chopped
- ¼ mug chives, sliced off
- 2 tbsp ghee
- 2 tbsp Dijon mustard

Instructions:

- Warm up a dish with 2 tbsp ghee over moderate heat, insert onion and a pair of garlic cloves, shake, prepare for three minutes and shift to a pot. In another pot, mix onion and garlic with salmon, chives, coconut flour, table salt, pepper, a pair of tbsp mustard and egg and shake well. Shape meatballs from the salmon mix, place on a baking sheet, introduce in the oven at 350 degrees F and bake for twenty-five minutes.
- Meanwhile, Warm up a dish with two tbsp ghee over moderate heat, insert 4 garlic cloves, shake and prepare for one minute. Insert coconut cream, a pair of tbsp Dijon mustard, lemon juice and zest and chives, shake and prepare for three minutes.

Lemon Cod with Arugula

Ingredients:

- 2 cod fillets
- 3 mug arugulas
- ½ mug black olives, pitted and sliced
- 2 tbsp capers
- 1 tablespoon olive oil
- Table salt and black pepper to the taste
- Juice of 1 lemon
- 1 garlic clove, sliced off

Instructions:

- Organize fish fillets in a heatproof dish, season with table salt, pepper, drizzle the oil and lemon juice, fling to coat, introduce in the oven at 450 degrees F and bake for 20 minutes. In your food processor, combine arugula with table salt, pepper, capers, olives and garlic and blend a bit. Organize fish on plates, top with arugula tapenade and serve.

Baked Halibut Balsamic Vinegar and Veggies

Ingredients:

- 1 tablespoon olive oil
- 2 halibut fillets
- 2 mugs baby spinach
- 1 red bell pepper, roughly sliced off
- 1 yellow bell pepper, roughly sliced off
- 1 tsp. balsamic vinegar
- Table salt and black pepper to the taste
- 1 tsp. cumin

Instructions:

- In a pot, combine bell peppers with table salt, pepper, half of the oil and the vinegar, fling to coat well and shift to a baking dish. Introduce in the oven at 400 degrees F and bake for 20 minutes. Warm up a dish with the rest of the oil over moderate heat, insert fish, season with table salt, pepper and cumin and brown on all sides.
- Take the baking dish out of the oven, insert spinach, shake gently and Distribute the whole combine between plates. Insert fish on the side, Garnish some more table salt and pepper and serve.

Fish Curry

Ingredients:

- 1 tsp. ginger, grated
- 1 tsp. curry grinding grains
- 1-inch turmeric root, grated
- ¼ mug cilantro
- 1 and ½ mugs coconut cream
- 3 garlic cloves, chopped
- ¼ tsp. cumin, ground
- 4 tbsp coconut oil
- 1 small red onion, sliced off
- 4 white fish fillets
- ½ tsp. mustard seeds
- Table salt and black pepper to the taste
- 2 green chilies, sliced off

Instructions:

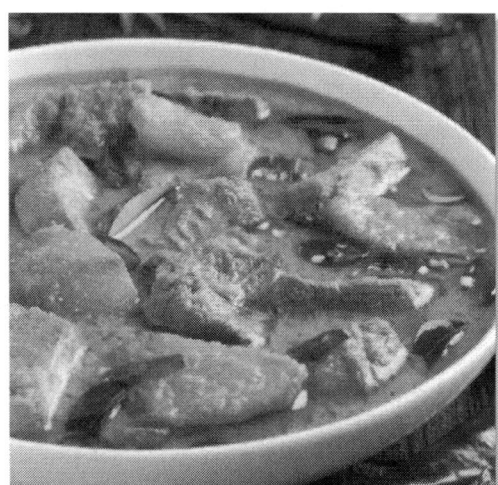

- Warm up a pot with half of the coconut oil over moderate heat, insert mustard seeds and prepare for two minutes. Insert ginger, onion and garlic, shake and prepare for 5 minutes. Insert turmeric, curry grinding grains, chilies and cumin, shake and prepare for 5 minutes additional.
- Insert coconut milk, table salt and pepper, shake, bring to a boil and prepare for 15 minutes. Heat up another dish with the remainder of the oil over moderate heat, insert fish, shake and prepare for 3 minutes. Insert this to the curry sauce, shake and prepare for 5 minutes additional. Insert cilantro, shake, distribute into pots and serve.

Green and Lean Shrimp

Ingredients:

- 2 tbsp lemon juice
- 2 tbsp garlic, chopped
- 1 tablespoon lemon zest
- 2 tbsp olive oil
- 1 tablespoon ghee
- 1-pound shrimp, peeled and deveined
- Table salt and black pepper to the taste

Instructions:

- Warm up a dish with the oil and the ghee over moderate immense heat, insert shrimp and prepare for 2 minutes. Insert garlic, shake and prepare for 4 minutes more. Insert lemon juice, lemon zest, table salt and pepper, shake, remove heat and serve.

Olive Barramundi

Ingredients:

- 2 barramundi fillets
- ¼ mug black olives, sliced off
- 1 tablespoon lemon zest
- 2 tbsp lemon zest
- Table salt and black pepper to the taste
- 2 tsp. olive oil
- 2 teaspoons Italian seasoning
- ¼ mug green olives, pitted and sliced off
- ¼ mug cherry tomatoes, sliced off
- 2 tbsp parsley, sliced off
- 1 tablespoon olive oil

Instructions:

- Rub fish with table salt, pepper, Italian seasoning and 2 teaspoons olive oil, shift to a baking dish and leave aside for now.
- Meanwhile, in a pot, combine tomatoes with all the olives, table salt, pepper, lemon zest and lemon juice, parsley and 1 tablespoon olive oil and fling everything well. Introduce fish in the oven at 400 degrees F and bake for 12 minutes. Distribute fish on plates, top with tomato relish and serve.

Garlic, Onion Shrimp

Ingredients:

1 tablespoon olive oil

- ½ mug cilantro, sliced off
- 1 tablespoon garlic, chopped
- ½ mug green onion, sliced off
- ½ tsp. red pepper flakes
- 1-pound shrimp, peeled and deveined
- Table salt and black pepper to the taste
- 4 cherry tomatoes, sliced off
- 2 mugs sugar snap peas, sliced lengthwise
- 1 red bell pepper, slice
- 10 ounces coconut milk
- 2 tbsp lime juice

Instructions:

- Warm up a dish with the oil over moderate immense heat, insert snap peas and shake-fry for 2 minutes. Insert pepper and prepare for 3 minutes more. Insert cilantro, garlic, green onions and pepper flakes, shake and prepare for 1 minute.
- Insert tomatoes and coconut milk, shake and simmer everything for 5 minutes. Insert shrimp and lime juice, shake and prepare for 3 minutes. Season with table salt and pepper, shake and serve warm.

Shrimp and Noodle Salad

Ingredients:

- Table salt and black pepper to the taste
- 1 tablespoon stevia
- 2 teaspoons fish sauce
- 1 cucumber, slice with a spiralizer
- ½ mug basil, sliced off
- ½ pound shrimp, already prepared, peeled and deveined
- 2 tbsp lime juice
- 2 teaspoons chili garlic sauce

Instructions:

- Put cucumber noodles on a paper towel, wrap up with another one and press well. Put into a pot and combine with basil, shrimp, table salt and pepper. In another pot, combine stevia with fish sauce, lime juice and chili sauce and whisk well. Insert this to shrimp salad, fling to coat well and serve.

Spicy Shrimp with Worcestershire Sauce

Ingredients:

- Juice of 1 lemon
- Table salt and black pepper to the taste
- 1 tsp. Creole seasoning
- ½ pound big shrimp, peeled and deveined
- 2 teaspoons Worcestershire sauce
- 2 teaspoons olive oil

Instructions:

- Organize shrimp in one layer in a baking dish, season with table salt and pepper and drizzle the oil. Insert Worcestershire sauce, lemon juice and Garnish Creole seasoning. Fling shrimp a bit, introduce in the oven, set it on the broiler and prepare for 8 minutes. Distribute between 2 plates and serve.

Shrimp Stew with Sriracha Sauce

Ingredients:

- ¼ mug red pepper, roasted and sliced off
- 14 ounces canned tomatoes, sliced off
- ¼ mug cilantro, sliced off
- 2 tbsp sriracha sauce
- ¼ mug yellow onion, sliced off
- ¼ mug olive oil
- 1 garlic clove, chopped
- 1 and ½ pounds shrimp, peeled and deveined
- 1 mug coconut milk
- Table salt and black pepper to the taste
- 2 tbsp lime juice

Instructions:

- Warm up a dish with the oil over moderate heat, insert onion, shake and prepare for 4 minutes. Insert peppers and garlic, shake and prepare for 4 minutes more. Insert cilantro, tomatoes and shrimp, shake and prepare until shrimp turn pink.
- Insert coconut milk and sriracha sauce, shake and bring to a gentle simmer. Insert table salt, pepper and lime juice, shake, shift to pots and serve.

Shrimp and Snow Peas Soup

Ingredients:

- ¼ mug coconut aminos
- 5 ounces canned bamboo shoots, sliced
- Black pepper to the taste
- ¼ tsp. fish sauce
- 1-pound shrimp, peeled and deveined
- ½ pound snow peas
- 4 scallions, sliced off
- 1 and ½ tbsp coconut oil
- 1 small ginger root, finely sliced off
- 8 mugs chicken stock
- 1 tablespoon sesame oil
- ½ tablespoon chili oil

Instructions:

- Warm up a pot with the coconut oil over moderate heat, insert scallions and ginger, shake and prepare for 2 minutes.
- Insert coconut aminos, stock, black pepper and fish sauce, shake and bring to a boil. Insert shrimp, snow peas and bamboo shoots, shake and prepare for 3 minutes. Insert sesame oil and warm chili oil, shake, distribute into pots and serve.

Mussels Dish
Ingredients:

- 1 tablespoon ghee
- A splash of lemon juice
- 2-pound mussels, debearded and scrubbed
- 2 garlic cloves, chopped

Instructions:

- Put some water in a pot, insert mussels, bring to a boil over moderate heat, prepare for 5 minutes, remove heat, remove unopened mussels and shift them to a pot.
- In another pot, combine ghee with garlic and lemon juice, whisk and Warm up in the microwave for 1 minute. Pour over mussels and serve them right away.

Baked Calamari, Avocado and Shrimp
Ingredients:

- 2 tbsp avocado, sliced off
- 1 tsp. tomato paste
- 1 tablespoon mayonnaise
- A splash of Worcestershire sauce
- 1 tsp. lemon juice
- 8 ounces calamari, slice into moderate rings
- 7 ounces shrimp, peeled and deveined
- 1 egg
- 3 tbsp coconut flour
- 1 tablespoon coconut oil
- 2 lemon slices
- Table salt and black pepper to the taste
- ½ tsp. turmeric

Instructions:

- During a pot, whisk the egg with coconut oil. Insert calamari rings and shrimp and fling to coat. In another pot, combine flour with table salt, pepper and turmeric and shake. Dredge calamari and shrimp during this mix, put everything on a lined baking sheet, introduce in the oven at 400 degrees F and bake for 10 minutes.
- Flip calamari and shrimp and bake for 10 minutes more. Meanwhile, in an exceedingly pot, mix avocado with mayo and tomato paste and mash employing a fork. Insert Worcestershire sauce, lemon juice, table salt and pepper and shake well. Distribute baked calamari and shrimp on plates and serve with the sauce and lemon juice on the aspect.

Green Octopus Salad

Ingredients:

- 3 ounces olive oil
- Table salt and black pepper to the taste
- 4 tbsp parsley, sliced off
- 21 ounces octopus, rinsed
- Juice of 1 lemon
- 4 celery stalks, sliced off

Instructions:

- Put the octopus in a pot, insert water to Wrap up, wrap up pot, bring to a boil over moderate heat, prepare for 40 minutes, drain and leave aside to cool down.
- Chop octopus and put it in a salad pot. Insert celery stalks, parsley, oil and lemon juice and fling well. Season with table salt and pepper, fling again and serve.

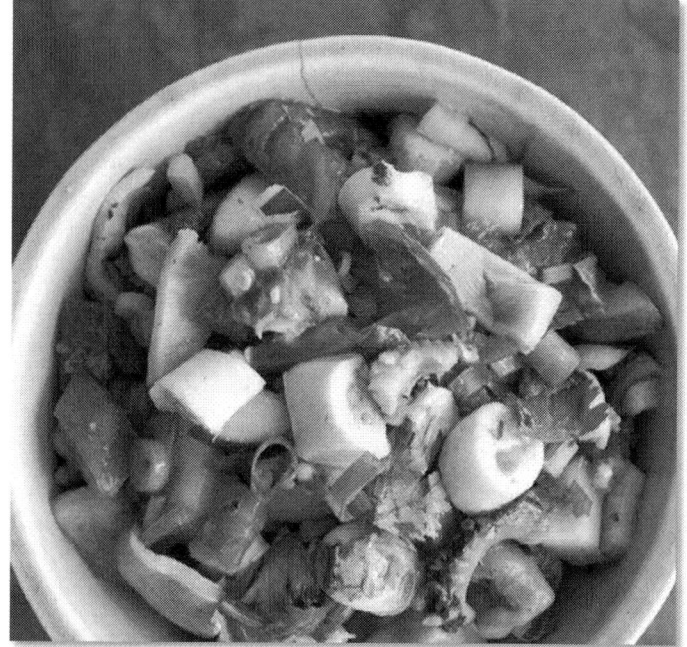

Stalks Clam Chowder

Ingredients:

- 2 mugs chicken stock
- 14 ounces canned baby clams
- 2 mugs whipping cream
- 1 mug celery stalks, sliced off
- Table salt and black pepper to the taste
- 1 tsp. thyme, ground
- 1 mug onion, sliced off
- 13 bacon slices, sliced off

Instructions:

- Warm up a dish over moderate heat, insert bacon slices, brown them and shift to a pot. Warm up the same dish over moderate heat, insert celery and onion, shake and prepare for 5 minutes.
- Shift everything to your Crockpot, also insert bacon, baby clams, table salt, pepper, stock, thyme and whipping cream, shake and prepare on Immense for 2 hours. Distribute into pots and serve.

Roasted Mahi Fillets and Salsa

Ingredients:

- 1 tsp. garlic, chopped
- 1 green bell pepper, sliced off
- ½ mug canned tomato salsa
- 2 tbsp kalamata olives, pitted and sliced off
- 2 mahi-mahi fillets
- ½ mug yellow onion, sliced off
- 4 teaspoons olive oil
- 1 tsp. Greek seasoning
- ¼ mug chicken stock
- Table salt and black pepper to the taste
- 2 tbsp feta cheese, crumbled

Instructions:

- Warm up a dish with a pair of teaspoons oil over moderate heat, insert bell pepper and onion, shake and prepare for 3 minutes. Insert Greek seasoning and garlic, shake and prepare for 1 minute more. Insert stock, olives and salsa, shake again and prepare until the mix thickens for five minutes. Shift to a pot and leave aside for currently.
- Warm up the dish again with the remainder of the oil over moderate heat, insert fish, season with table salt and pepper and prepare for two minutes. Flip prepares for 2 minutes a lot of and shift to a baking dish. Spoon salsa over fish, introduce within the oven and bake at 425 degrees F for six minutes. Garnish feta on prime and serve warm.

Flounder and Shrimp

Ingredients:

- 2 teaspoons garlic grinding grains
- Table salt and black pepper to the taste
- ½ tsp. allspice, ground
- 1 tsp. oregano, dried
- 2 teaspoons onion grinding grains
- 2 teaspoons thyme, dried
- 2 teaspoons sweet paprika
- A pinch of cayenne pepper
- ¼ tsp. nutmeg, ground
- 1 tsp. Tabasco sauce
- Table salt and black pepper to the taste
- 4 flounder fillets
- 2 tbsp ghee
- ¼ tsp. cloves
- 1 celery stick, sliced off
- 2 tbsp coconut flour

- 1 tomato, sliced off
- 4 garlic cloves, chopped
- 8 ounces shrimp, peeled, deveined and sliced off
- 2 mugs chicken stock
- 1 tablespoon coconut milk
- A pinch of cinnamon grinding grains
- 2 shallots, sliced off
- 1 tablespoon ghee
- 8 ounces bacon, sliced
- 1 green bell pepper, sliced off
- A handful parsley, sliced off

Instructions:

- In a pot, combine paprika with thyme, garlic and onion grinding grains, table salt, pepper, oregano, allspice, cayenne pepper, cloves, nutmeg and cinnamon and shake. Reserve two tbsp of this combine rub the flounder with the rest and leave aside. Warm up a dish over moderate heat, insert bacon, shake and prepare for 6 minutes. Insert celery, bell pepper, shallots and 1 tablespoon ghee, shake and prepare for 4 minutes. Insert tomato and garlic, shake and prepare for 4 minutes.
- Insert coconut flour and reserved seasoning, shake and prepare for 2 minutes additional. Insert chicken stock and convey to a simmer.
- Meanwhile, Warm up a dish with 2 tbsp ghee over moderate immense heat, insert fish, prepare for two minutes, flip and slice for two minutes more. Insert shrimp to the dish with the stock, shake and prepare for two minutes. Insert parsley, table salt, pepper, coconut milk and Tabasco sauce, shake and take away heat. Distribute fish on plates, top with the shrimp sauce and serve.

Green Shrimp Salad
Ingredients:

- 2 tbsp olive oil
- 3 tbsp parsley, sliced off
- 2 teaspoons mint, sliced off
- 1 tablespoon tarragon, sliced off
- 1 tablespoon lemon juice
- 2 tbsp mayonnaise
- 1-pound shrimp, peeled and deveined
- Table salt and black pepper to the taste
- 2 tbsp lime juice
- 3 endives, leaves separated
- 1 tsp. lime zest
- ½ mug sour cream

Instructions:

- In a pot, combine shrimp with table salt, pepper and the olive oil, fling to coat and Scatter them on a lined baking sheet. Introduce shrimp in the oven at 400 degrees F and bake for 10 minutes. Insert lime juice, fling them to coat again and leave aside for now.
- In a pot, combine mayo with sour cream, lime zest, lemon juice, table salt, pepper, tarragon, mint and parsley and shake very well. Chop shrimp insert to salad dressing, fling to coat everything and spoon into endive leaves. Serve right away.

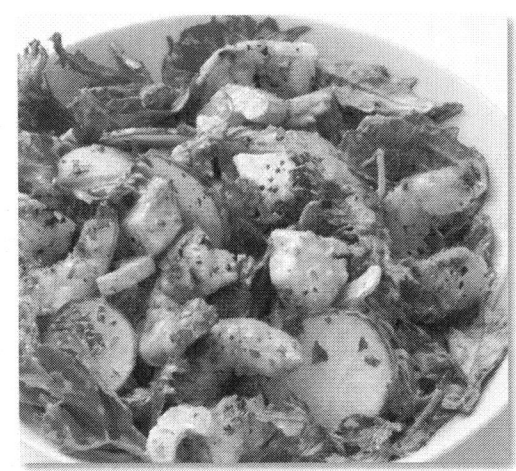

Lean and Green Oysters

Ingredients:

- Zest from 1 lime
- ¼ mug olive oil
- ¼ mug cilantro, sliced off
- ¼ mug scallions, sliced off
- 2 tbsp ketchup
- 1 Serrano chili pepper, sliced off
- 1 mug tomato juice
- ½ tsp. ginger, grated
- ¼ tsp. garlic, chopped
- 12 oysters, shucked
- Juice of 1 lemon
- Juice from 1 orange
- Zest from 1 orange
- Juice from 1 lime
- Table salt to the taste

Instructions:

- In a pot, combine lemon juice, orange juice, orange zest, lime juice and zest, ketchup, chili pepper, tomato juice, ginger, garlic, oil, scallions, cilantro and table salt and shake well. Spoon this into oysters and serve them.

Salmon Rolls

Ingredients:

- 4 ounces cream cheese
- 1 cucumber, sliced
- 2 nori seeds
- 1 small avocado, pitted, peeled and finely sliced off
- 6 ounces smoked salmon. Sliced

- 1 tsp. wasabi paste
- Pickled ginger for serving

Instructions:

- Put nori sheets on a sushi mat. Distribute salmon slices on them and also avocado and cucumber slices. In a pot, combine cream cheese with wasabi paste and shake well. Scatter this over cucumber slices, roll your nori sheets, press well, slice each into 6 pieces and serve with pickled ginger.

Salmon Skewers
Ingredients:

- ½ green bell pepper slice in chunks
- ½ orange bell pepper slice in chunks
- Juice from 1 lemon
- 12 ounces salmon fillet, cubed
- 1 red onion, slice into chunks
- ½ red bell pepper slice in chunks
- Table salt and black pepper to the taste
- A drizzle of olive oil

Instructions:

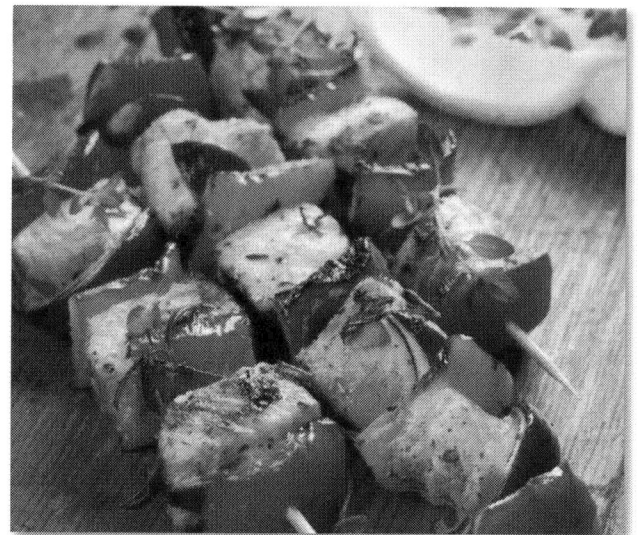

- Thread skewers with onion, red, green and orange pepper and salmon cubes. Season them with table salt and pepper, drizzle oil and lemon juice and Put them on preheated grill over moderate immense heat. Prepare for 4 minutes on each side, distribute between plates and serve.

Grilled Basil Shrimp
Ingredients:

- ½ mug basil leaves
- 1 tablespoon pine nuts, toasted
- 2 tbsp parmesan, grated
- 1-pound shrimp, peeled and deveined
- 1 tablespoon lemon juice
- 1 garlic clove, chopped
- 2 tbsp olive oil
- Table salt and black pepper to the taste

Instructions:

- In your food processor, combine parmesan with basil, garlic, pine nuts, oil, table salt, pepper and lemon juice and blend well.
- Shift this to a pot, insert shrimp, fling to coat and leave aside for 20 minutes. Thread skewers with marinated shrimp, put them on preheated grill over moderate immense heat, prepare for 3 minutes, flip and prepare for 3 more minutes. Organize on plates and serve.

Lean Calamari Salad
Ingredients:

- 3 green onions, sliced off
- 1 tablespoon balsamic vinegar
- Table salt and black pepper to the taste
- Juice of 1 lemon
- 6 pounds calamari hoods, tentacles reserved
- 2 long red chilies, sliced off
- 2 small red chilies, sliced off
- 2 garlic cloves, chopped
- 3.5 ounces olive oil
- 3 ounces rocket for serving

Instructions:

- In a pot, combine long red chilies with little red chilies, green onions, vinegar, of the oil, garlic, table salt, pepper and lemon juice and shake well. Put calamari and tentacles in a pot, season with table salt and pepper, drizzle the rest of the oil, fling to coat and Put-on preheated grill over moderate immense heat.
- Prepare for 2 minutes on each aspect and shift to the chili marinade you've got made. Fling to coat and leave aside for 30 minutes. Organize rocket on plates, prime with calamari and its marinade and serve.

Kalamata Olives Salad
Ingredients:

- ¾ mug olive oil
- Table salt and black pepper to the taste
- Juice from 2 lemons
- 1 mug kalamata olives, pitted and sliced off
- 6 tbsp capers
- ½ tsp. red chili flakes
- 1 escarole head, leaves separated
- 4 garlic cloves, chopped
- 2 celery ribs, sliced off
- 2 mugs jarred pimiento peppers, sliced off
- 2 pounds table salt cod

- 1 mug parsley, sliced off

Instructions:

- Put cod in a pot, insert water to Wrap up, bring to a boil over moderate heat, boil for 20 minutes, drain and slice into moderate chunks. Put cod in a salad pot, insert peppers, parsley, olives, capers, celery, garlic, lemon juice, table salt, pepper, olive oil and chili flakes and fling to coat. Organize escarole leaves on a platter, insert cod salad and serve.

Sardines Salad

Ingredients:

- ½ tablespoon mustard
- Table salt and black pepper to the taste
- 5 ounces canned sardines in oil
- 1 tbsp lemon juice
- 1 small cucumber, sliced off

Instructions:

- Drain sardines, put them in a pot and mash using a fork. Insert table salt, pepper, cucumber, lemon juice and mustard, shake well and serve cold.

Tuna and Chimichurri Sauce

Ingredients:

2 tbsp parsley, sliced off

- 2 tbsp basil, sliced off
- 1 jalapeno pepper, sliced off
- A pinch of cayenne pepper
- 3 garlic cloves, chopped
- 2 avocados, pitted, peeled and sliced
- 6 ounces baby arugula
- 1-pound sushi grade tuna steak
- Table salt and black pepper to the taste
- 1 tsp. red pepper flakes
- ½ mug cilantro, sliced off
- 1/3 mug olive oil
- 2 tbsp olive oil
- 1 small red onion, sliced off
- 3 tablespoon balsamic vinegar
- 1 tsp. thyme, sliced off

Instructions:

- In a pot, combine 1/3 mug oil with jalapeno, vinegar, onion, cilantro, basil, garlic, parsley, pepper flakes, thyme, cayenne, table salt and pepper, whisk well and leave aside for now. Warm up a dish with the remainder of the oil over moderate immense heat, insert tuna, season with table salt and pepper, prepare for 2 minutes on each aspect, shift to a   board, leave aside to chill down a bit and slice.
- Mix arugula with 0.5 of the chimichurri mix you've got made and fling to coat. Distribute arugula on plates, high with tuna slices, drizzle the remainder of the chimichurri sauce and serve with avocado slices on the side.

Salmon Bites and Chili Sauce

Ingredients:

- 1/3 mug coconut flour
- 3 tbsp coconut oil
- For the sauce:
- ¼ tsp. agar and
- 3 garlic cloves, sliced off
- ¾ mug water
- 1 and ¼ mugs coconut, desiccated and unsweetened
- 1-pound salmon, cubed
- 1 egg
- Table salt and black pepper
- 1 tablespoon water
- 4 Thai red chilies, sliced off
- ¼ mug balsamic vinegar
- ½ mug stevia
- A pinch of table salt

Instructions:

- In an exceedingly pot, mix flour with table salt and pepper and shake. In another pot, whisk egg and 1 tablespoon water. Put the coconut during a third pot. Dip salmon cubes in flour, egg and then in coconut and Put them on a plate.
- Warm up a dish with the coconut oil over moderate immense heat, insert salmon bites, prepare for three minutes on each aspect and shift them to paper towels. Warm up a dish with ¾ mug water over immense heat, Garnish agar chilies, sliced and bring to a boil. Prepare for 3 minutes and remove heat.
- In your blender, mix garlic with chilies, vinegar, stevia and a pinch of table salt and blend well. Shift this to a tiny dish and Warm up over moderate immense heat. Shake, insert agar mix and prepare for three minutes. Serve your salmon bites with chili sauce on the side.

Discrete Olive Clams

Ingredients:

- 2 garlic cloves, chopped
- 1 bottle infused cider
- Table salt and black pepper to the taste
- Juice of ½ lemon
- 1 small green apple, sliced off
- 2 pounds clams, scrubbed
- 3 ounces discrete
- 1 tablespoon olive oil
- 3 tbsp ghee
- 2 thyme springs, sliced off

Instructions:

- Heat up a dish with the oil over moderate immense heat, insert discrete, brown for three minutes and reduce tempera to moderate. Insert ghee, garlic, table salt, pepper and shallot, shake and prepare for three minutes.
- Expand heat again, insert cider, shake well and prepare for 1 minute. Insert clams and thyme, Wrap up dish and simmer for 5 minutes. Remove unopened clams, insert lemon juice and apple pieces, shake and Distribute into pots. Serve heat.

Scallops and Roasted Grapes

Ingredients:

- 2 mugs spinach
- 1 mug chicken stock
- 1 Romanesco lettuce head
- 1 and ½ mugs red grapes, slice in halves
- 1-pound scallops
- 3 tbsp olive oil
- 1 shallot, sliced off
- 3 garlic cloves, chopped
- ¼ mug walnuts, toasted and sliced off
- 1 tablespoon ghee
- Table salt and black pepper to the taste

Instructions:

- Put Romanesco in your food processor, blend and shift to a pot. Heat up a dish with two tbsp oil over moderate immense heat, insert shallot and garlic, shake and prepare for 1 minute. Insert Romanesco, spinach and 1 mug stock, shake, prepare for 3 minutes, mix using an immersion blender and take away heat.
- Warm up another dish with one tablespoon oil and also the ghee over moderate immense heat, insert scallops, season with table salt and pepper, prepare for two minutes, flip and sear

for one minute more. Distribute Romanesco combine on plates, insert scallops on the aspect, high with walnuts and grapes and serve.

Chicken Cayenne Pepper Stuffed Avocado
Ingredients:

- 1 and ½ mugs chicken, prepared and shredded
- Table salt and black pepper to the taste
- ¼ tsp. cayenne pepper
- ½ tsp. onion grinding grains
- ½ tsp. garlic grinding grains
- 2 avocados, slice in halves and pitted
- ¼ mug mayonnaise
- 1 tsp. thyme, dried
- 2 tbsp cream cheese
- 1 tsp. paprika
- Table salt and black pepper to the taste
- 2 tbsp lemon juice

Instructions:

- Scoop the insides of your avocado halves and put the flesh in a pot. Leave avocado mugs aside for now. Insert chicken to avocado flesh and shake.
- Also insert mayo, thyme, cream cheese, cayenne, onion, garlic, paprika, table salt, pepper and lemon juice and shake well. Stuff avocados with chicken combine and serve.

Oysters and Monterey Jack cheese
Ingredients:

- ¼ mug red onion, finely sliced off
- Table salt and black pepper to the taste
- ½ mug Monterey Jack cheese, shredded
- 18 oysters, scrubbed
- A handful cilantro, sliced off
- 2 tomatoes, sliced off
- 1 jalapeno pepper, sliced off
- 2 limes, slice into wedges
- Juice from 1 lime

Instructions:

- In a pot, mix onion with jalapeno, cilantro, tomatoes, table salt, pepper and lime juice and shake well. Put oysters on preheated grill over moderate immense heat, finish grill and prepare for seven minutes till they open. Shift opened oysters to a heatproof dish and remove unopened ones.

- Top oysters with cheese and introduce in preheated broiler for one minute. Organize oysters on a platter, high every with tomatoes combine you've created earlier and serve with lime wedges on the side.

Grilled Squid and Black Pepper

Ingredients:

- 2 avocados, pitted, peeled and sliced off
- Some coriander springs, sliced off
- 2 red chilies, sliced off
- 2 moderate squids, tentacles separated, and tubes scored lengthwise
- A drizzle of olive oil
- Juice from 1 lime
- Table salt and black pepper to the taste
- 1 tomato, sliced off
- 1 red onion, sliced off
- Juice from 2 limes

Instructions:

- Season squid and squid tentacles with table salt, pepper, drizzle some olive oil and massage well. Put on preheated grill over moderate immense heat score aspect down and prepare for 2 minutes. Flip and prepare for 2 minutes additional and shift to a pot. Insert juice from 1 lime, fling to coat and keep warm.
- Put avocado in an exceedingly pot and mash employing a fork. Insert coriander, chilies, tomato, onion and juice from 2 limes and shake well everything. Distribute squid on plates, high with guacamole and serve.

Chicken Wings and Tasty Mint Sauce

Ingredients:

- 1 tablespoon paprika
- A pinch of cayenne pepper
- Table salt and black pepper to the taste
- 2 tbsp olive oil
- Juice of ½ lime
- 1 mug mint leaves
- 1 small ginger piece, sliced off
- ¾ mug cilantro
- 18 chicken wings, slice in halves
- 1 tablespoon turmeric
- 1 tablespoon cumin, ground
- 1 tablespoon ginger, grated
- 1 tablespoon coriander, ground
- 1 tablespoon olive oil

- 1 tablespoon water
- Table salt and black pepper to the taste
- 1 Serrano pepper

Instructions:

- In a pot, combine 1 tablespoon ginger with cumin, coriander, paprika, turmeric, table salt, pepper, cayenne and a pair of tbsp oil and shake well. Insert chicken wings pieces to this mix, fling to coat well and keep within the fridge for twenty minutes.
- Warm up your grill over immense heat, insert marinated wings, prepare for twenty-five minutes, turning them sometimes and shift to a pot. In your blender, combine mint with cilantro, 1 tiny ginger items, juice from ½ lime, one tablespoon olive oil, table salt, pepper, water and Serrano pepper and mix terribly well. Serve your chicken wings with this sauce on the side.

Chicken Kofta
Ingredients:

- ¼ mug cheddar cheese, grated
- 1 tablespoon dry ranch seasoning
- ¼ mug warm sauce+ some more for serving
- 1-pound chicken meat, ground
- Table salt and black pepper to the taste
- 2 tbsp ranch dressing
- ½ mug almond flour
- 1 egg

Instructions:

- In a pot, combine chicken meat with table salt, pepper, ranch dressing, flour, dry ranch seasoning, cheddar cheese, warm sauce and the egg and Shake very well. Shape 9 meatballs put them all on a lined baking sheet and bake at 500 degrees F for 15 minutes. Serve chicken meatballs with warm sauce on the side.

Tasty Grilled Chicken Niblets
Ingredients:

- 1 jalapeno pepper, sliced off
- 3 tbsp coconut oil
- Table salt and black pepper to the taste
- Lime wedges for serving
- 2 pounds wings
- Juice from 1 lime
- 1 handful cilantro, sliced off
- 2 garlic cloves, chopped
- Ranch dip for serving

Instructions:

- In a pot, combine lime juice with cilantro, garlic, jalapeno, coconut oil, table salt and pepper and whisk well. Insert chicken wings, fling to coat and keep in the fridge for 2 hours. Put chicken wings on your preheated grill over moderate immense heat and prepare for 7 minutes on each side.
- Serve these amazing chicken wings with ranch did and lime wedges on the side.

Onion Baked Chicken

Ingredients:

- 4 bacon strips
- 1-ounce coconut aminos
- 2 tbsp coconut oil
- 4 ounces cheddar cheese, grated
- 4 chicken breasts
- 3 green onions, sliced off
- 4 ounces ranch dressing

Instructions:

- Heat up a dish with the oil over immense heat, insert chicken breasts, prepare for seven minutes, flip and prepare for seven a lot of minutes. Meanwhile, heat up another dish over moderate immense heat, insert bacon, prepare till it's crispy, shift to paper towels, drain grease and crumble.
- Shift chicken breast to a baking dish, insert coconut aminos, crumbled bacon, cheese and inexperienced onions on high, introduce in your oven, set on broiler and prepare at an immense tempera for five minutes more. Distribute between plates and serve heat.

Special Iranian Chicken

Ingredients:

- ½ mug Italian olives, pitted and sliced off
- 4 anchovy fillets, sliced off
- 1 tablespoon capers, sliced off
- 1-pound tomatoes, sliced off
- ¼ mug olive oil
- 1 red onion, sliced off
- 4 chicken breasts, skinless and boneless
- 4 garlic cloves, chopped
- Table salt and black pepper to the taste
- ½ tsp. red chili flakes

Instructions:

- Season chicken with table salt and pepper and rub with half of the oil. Put into a dish that you have heated over immense tempera, prepare for two minutes, flip and prepare for two minutes more. Introduce chicken breasts within the oven at 450 degrees F and bake for eight minutes. Take chicken out of the oven and Distribute between plates.

- Warm up the same dish with the rest of the oil over moderate heat, insert capers, onion, garlic, olives, anchovies, chili flakes and capers, shake and prepare for 1 minute. Insert table salt, pepper and tomatoes, shake and prepare for two minutes more. Drizzle this over chicken breasts and serve.

Lemon Chicken

Ingredients:

- Zest from 2 lemons
- Lemon rinds from 2 lemons
- 1 whole chicken, slice into moderate pieces
- Table salt and black pepper to the taste
- Juice from 2 lemons

Instructions:

- Put chicken pieces in a baking dish, season with table salt and pepper to the taste and drizzle lemon juice. Fling to coat well, insert lemon zest and lemon rinds, introduce in the oven at 375 degrees F and bake for 45 minutes.
- Remove lemon rinds, distribute chicken between plates, drizzle sauce from the baking dish over it and serve.

Orange Glazed Salmon

Ingredients:

- 2 lemons, sliced
- ¼ mug red orange juice
- 1 tsp. coconut oil
- 1-pound wild salmon, skinless and cubed
- ¼ mug balsamic vinegar
- 1/3 mug orange marmalade, no sugar inserted

Instructions:

- Warm up a pot over moderate warmth, embed vinegar, squeezed orange and jelly, shake well, bring to a stew for 1 moment, lessen gum-based paint, plan until it thickens a piece and eliminate heat. Arrange salmon and lemon cuts on sticks and brush them on one side with the orange coating.
- Brush your kitchen flame broil with coconut oil and Warm up over moderate warmth. Put salmon kebabs on flame broil with coated side down and get ready for 4 minutes. Flip kebabs brush them with the remainder of the orange coating and plan for 4 minutes more. Serve immediately.

Chicken Fajitas

Ingredients:

- 2 tbsp lime juice
- Table salt and black pepper to the taste
- 1 yellow onion, sliced
- 1 tablespoon cilantro, sliced off
- 1 avocado, pitted, peeled and sliced
- 2 limes, slice into wedges
- 1 tsp. sweet paprika
- 2 tbsp coconut oil
- 1 tsp. coriander, ground
- 2 pounds chicken breasts, skinless, boneless and slice into strips
- 1 tsp. garlic grinding grains
- 1 tsp. chili grinding grains
- 2 teaspoons cumin
- 1 green bell pepper, sliced
- 1 red bell pepper, sliced

Instructions:

- In a pot, mix lime juice with chili grinding grains, cumin, table salt, pepper, garlic grinding grains, paprika and coriander and shake. Insert chicken items and fling to coat well. Warm up a dish with 0.5 of the oil over moderate immense heat, insert chicken, prepare for 3 minutes on every facet and shift to a pot.
- Warm up the dish with the remainder of the oil over moderate heat, insert onion and all bell peppers, shake and prepare for six minutes. Return chicken to dish, insert a lot of table salt and pepper, shake and Distribute between plates. Top with avocado, lime wedges and cilantro and serve.

Skillet Chicken Tim menses and Mushrooms

Ingredients:

- ½ tsp. onion grinding grains
- ½ tsp. garlic grinding grains
- ½ mug water
- 1 tsp. Dijon mustard
- 4 chicken
- 2 mugs mushrooms, sliced
- ¼ mug ghee
- Table salt and black pepper to the taste
- 1 tablespoon tarragon, sliced off

Instructions:

- Warm up a dish with 0.5 of the ghee over moderate immense heat, insert chicken, season them with table salt, pepper, garlic grinding grains and onion grinding grains, prepare them for three minutes on every facet and shift to a pot.
- Warm up the identical dish with the remainder of the ghee over moderate immense heat, insert mushrooms, shake and prepare for 5 minutes. Insert mustard and water and shake well. Return chicken pieces to the dish, shake, finish and prepare for fifteen minutes. Insert tarragon, shake, prepare for 5 minutes, distribute between plates and serve.

Chicken and Olives Tapenade

Ingredients:

- ½ mug olives tapenade
- For the tapenade:
- 1 mug black olives, pitted
- Table salt and black pepper to the taste
- 1 chicken breast slice into 4 pieces
- 2 tbsp coconut oil
- 3 garlic cloves, crushed
- 2 tbsp olive oil
- ¼ mug parsley, sliced off
- 1 tbsp lemon juice

Instructions:

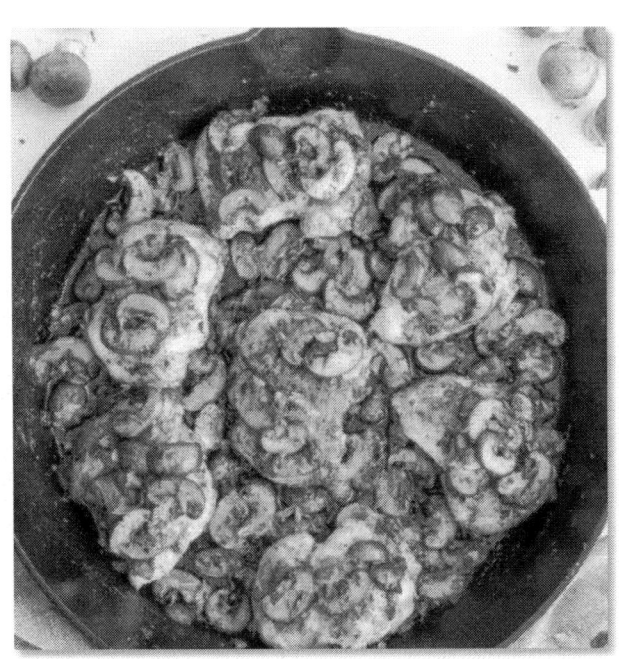

- In your food processor, combine olives with table salt, pepper, 2 tbsp olive oil, lemon juice and parsley, blend very well and shift to a pot. Warm up a dish with the coconut oil over moderate heat, insert garlic, shake and prepare for 2 minutes. Insert chicken pieces and prepare for 4 minutes on each side.
- Distribute chicken on plates and top with the olive's tapenade.

Duck Breast

Ingredients:

- ½ tsp. orange extract
- Table salt and black pepper to the taste
- 1 mug baby spinach
- ¼ tsp. sage
- 1 moderate duck breast, skin scored
- 1 tablespoon swerve
- 1 tablespoon heavy cream

- 2 tbsp ghee

Instructions:

- Warm up a dish with the ghee over moderate warmth. When it dissolves, embed turn and shake until ghee tans. Addition oranges concentrate and sage, shake and get ready for 2 minutes more.
- Supplement substantial cream and shake once more. In the interim, Warm up another dish over moderate massive warmth, embed duck bosom, skin side down, plan for 4 minutes, flip and get ready for an additional 3 minutes.
- Pour orange sauce over duck bosom, shake and plan for a couple of moments more. Addition spinach to the dish where you've made the sauce, shake and plan for 1 moment. Take duck off warmth, cut duck bosom and Organize on a plate. Sprinkle the orange sauce on top and present with the spinach as an afterthought.

Turkey Paprika Pie

Ingredients:

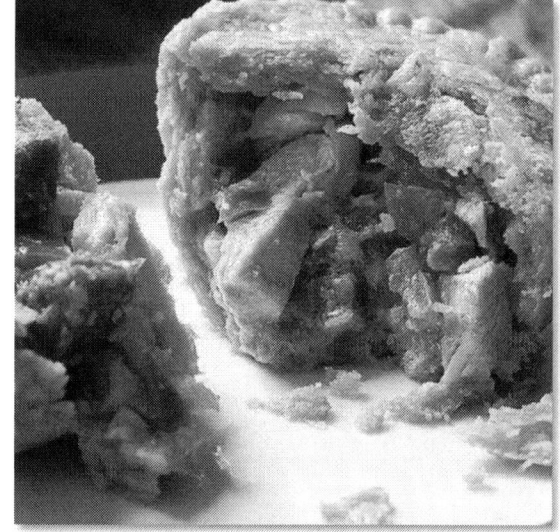

- ½ mug butternut squash, peeled and sliced off
- ½ mug cheddar cheese, shredded
- ¼ tsp. paprika
- ¼ tsp. garlic grinding grains
- ¼ tsp. xanthan gum
- 2 mugs turkey stock
- 1 mug turkey meat, prepared and shredded
- Table salt and black pepper to the taste
- 1 tsp. thyme, sliced off
- ½ mug kale, sliced off
- Preparing spray
- ¼ mug ghee
- ¼ tsp. xanthan gum
- 2 mugs almond flour
- A pinch of table salt
- 1 egg
- ¼ mug cheddar cheese

Instructions:

- Warm up a pot with the stock over moderate warmth. Addition squash and turkey meat shake and plan for 10 minutes. Addition garlic crushing grains, kale, thyme, paprika, table salt, pepper and ½ mug cheddar and shake well. In a pot, join ¼ tsp. thickener with ½ mug stock from the pot, shake well and supplement everything to the pot. Eliminate warmth and leave aside for the present.
- In a pot, consolidate flour with ¼ tsp. thickener and a spot of table salt and shake. Addition ghee, egg and ¼ mug cheddar and shake everything until you acquire your pie covering batter. Shape a ball and keep in the cooler for the present. Splash a heating dish with getting

ready shower and Scatter pie filling on the base. Move mixture to a working surface, fold into a circle and top loading up with this.

- Press well and seal edges, present in the stove at 350 degrees F and prepare for 35 minutes. Leave the pie to chill off a piece and serve.

Turkey Parsley Soup
Ingredients:

- 6 mugs turkey stock
- Table salt and black pepper to the taste
- ¼ mug parsley, sliced off
- 3 mugs baked spaghetti squash, sliced off
- 3 celery stalks, sliced off
- 1 yellow onion, sliced off
- 1 tablespoon ghee
- 3 mugs turkey, prepared and shredded

Instructions:

- Warm up a pot with the ghee over moderate immense heat, insert celery and onion, shake and prepare for 5 minutes. Insert parsley, stock, turkey meat, table salt and pepper, shake and prepare for 20 minutes.
- Insert spaghetti squash, shake and prepare turkey soup for 10 minutes more. Distribute into pots and serve.

Turkey Chili
Ingredients:

- 1 tablespoon canned chipotle peppers, sliced off
- ½ tsp. garlic grinding grains
- ½ mug salsa Verde
- 1 tsp. coriander, ground
- 2 teaspoons cumin, ground
- 4 mugs turkey meat, prepared and shredded
- 2 mugs squash, sliced off
- 6 mugs chicken stock
- Table salt and black pepper to the taste
- ¼ mug sour cream
- 1 tablespoon cilantro, sliced off

Instructions:

- Warm up a dish with the stock over moderate heat. Insert squash, shake and prepare for 10 minutes. Insert turkey, chipotles, garlic grinding grains, salsa Verde, cumin, coriander, table salt and pepper, shake and prepare for 10 minutes.

- Insert sour cream, shake, remove heat and Distribute into pots. Top with some sliced off cilantro and serve.

Turkey and Tomato Curry

Ingredients:

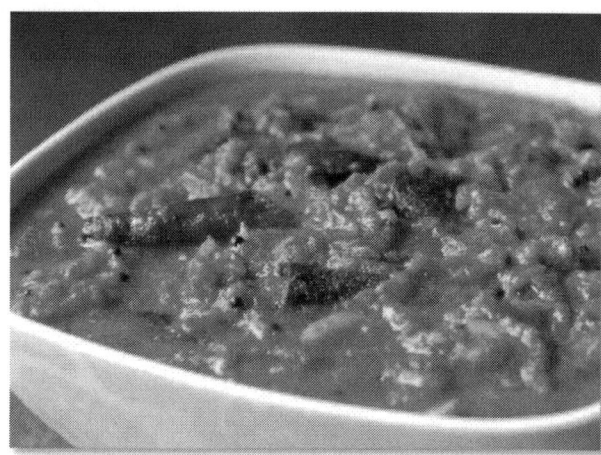

- 2 garlic cloves, chopped
- 2 yellow onions, sliced
- 1 tablespoon coriander, ground
- 2 tbsp ginger, grated
- 1 tbsp turmeric
- 1 tablespoon cumin, ground
- 18 ounces turkey meat, chopped
- 3 ounces spinach
- 20 ounces canned tomatoes, sliced off
- 2 tbsp coconut oil
- 2 tbsp coconut cream
- Table salt and black pepper to the taste
- 2 tbsp chili grinding grains

Instructions:

- Warm up a dish with the coconut oil over moderate heat, insert onion, shake and prepare for 5 minutes. Insert ginger and garlic, shake and prepare for 1 minute. Insert tomatoes, table salt, pepper, coriander, cumin, turmeric and chili grinding grains and shake.
- Insert coconut cream, shake and prepare for 10 minutes. Blend using an immersion blender and combine with spinach and turkey meat. Bring to a simmer, prepare for 15 minutes more and serve.

Green Cranberry Salad

Ingredients:

- 3 kiwis, peeled and sliced
- ¼ mug cranberries
- 1 mug cranberry sauce
- 4 mugs romaine lettuce leaves, torn
- 2 mugs turkey breast, prepared and cubed
- 1 orange, peeled and slice into small segments
- 1 red apple, cored and sliced off
- 3 tbsp walnuts, sliced off
- 1 mug orange juice

Instructions:

- In a salad pot, combine lettuce with turkey, orange segments, apple pieces, cranberries and walnut and fling to coat. In another pot, combine cranberry sauce and orange juice and shake. Drizzle this over turkey salad, fling to coat and serve with kiwis on top.

Spinach Chicken Breast

Ingredients:

- 4 ounces cream cheese, soft
- 3 ounces feta cheese, crumbled
- 1 garlic clove, chopped
- 8 ounces spinach, prepared and sliced off
- 3 chicken breasts
- Table salt and black pepper to the taste
- 1 tablespoon coconut oil

Instructions:

- In a pot, combine feta cheese with cream cheese, spinach, table salt, pepper and therefore the garlic and shake well. Put chicken breasts on a working surface, slice a pocket in each, stuff them with the spinach combine and season them with table salt and pepper to the taste.
- Warm up a dish with the oil over moderate immense heat, insert stuffed chicken, prepare for five minutes on every side and then introduce everything within the oven at 450 degrees F. Bake for 10 minutes, distribute between plates and serve.

Chicken and Mustard Sauce

Ingredients:

- 1 tablespoon olive oil
- 1 and ½ mugs chicken stock
- 3 chicken breasts, skinless and boneless
- 8 bacon strips, sliced off
- 1/3 mug Dijon mustard
- Table salt and black pepper to the taste
- 1 mug yellow onion, sliced off
- ¼ tsp. sweet paprika

Instructions:

- In a pot, consolidate paprika with mustard, table salt and pepper and shake well. Disperse this on chicken bosoms and back rub. Warm up a dish over moderate colossal warmth, embed bacon, shake, plan until it tans and move to a plate. Warm up a similar dish with the oil over moderate massive warmth, embed chicken bosoms, plan for 2 minutes on each side and furthermore move to a plate.
- Warm up the dish indeed over moderate tremendous warmth, embed stock, shake and bring to a stew. Supplement bacon and onions, table salt and pepper and shake. Return chicken to

dish also, shake delicately and stew over moderate warmth for 20 minutes, turning meat midway. Appropriate chicken on plates, sprinkle the sauce over it and serve.

Amazing Salsa Chicken

Ingredients:

- 6 chicken breasts, skinless and boneless
- 1 mug cheddar cheese, shredded
- Vegetable preparing spray
- 2 mugs jarred salsa
- Table salt and black pepper to the taste

Instructions:

- Spray a baking dish with preparing oil, put chicken breasts on it, season with table salt and pepper and pour salsa all over. Introduce in the oven at 425 degrees F and bake for 1 hour. Scatter cheese and bake for 15 minutes more. Distribute between plates and serve.

Asian Chicken

Ingredients:

- 1 red onion, sliced
- 2 tbsp garlic, chopped
- 1 tablespoon balsamic vinegar
- 2 teaspoons oregano, dried
- Some sliced off parsley for serving
- 2 mugs cherry tomatoes, halved
- 4 chicken
- 8 ounces mushrooms, sliced off
- 1-pound Italian sausage, sliced off
- 2 tbsp avocado oil
- 6 cherry peppers, sliced off
- 1 red bell pepper, sliced off
- Table salt and black pepper to the taste
- ½ mug chicken stock

Instructions:

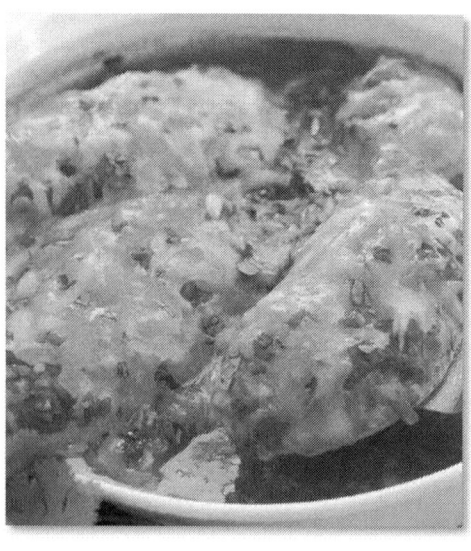

- Warm up a dish with half of the oil over moderate warmth, embed hotdogs, shake, earthy colored for a couple of moments and move to a plate.
- Warm up the dish again with the remainder of the oil over moderate warmth, embed chicken, season with table salt and pepper, get ready for 3 minutes on each side and move to a plate. Warm up the dish again over

moderate warmth, embed cherry peppers, mushrooms, onion and chime pepper, shake and get ready for 4 minutes.

- Addition garlic, shake and get ready for 2 minutes. Addition stock, vinegar, table salt, pepper, oregano and cherry tomatoes and shake. Addition chicken pieces and frankfurters ones, shake tenderly, move everything to the broiler at 400 degrees and heat for 30 minutes. Trimming parsley, appropriate among plates and serve.

Chicken Casserole
Ingredients:

- ¼ mug parmesan, grated
- ½ tsp. garlic grinding grains
- 1 and ½ teaspoons parsley, dried
- ½ tsp. basil, dried
- 4 tbsp avocado oil
- 1 and ½ pounds chicken breast, skinless and boneless and cubed
- Table salt and black pepper to the taste
- 1 egg
- 1 mug almond flour
- 4 mugs spaghetti squash, already prepared
- 6 ounces mozzarella, shredded
- 1 and ½ mugs marinara sauce
- Fresh basil, sliced off for serving

Instructions:

- In a pot, consolidate almond flour with pram, table salt, pepper, garlic granulating grains and 1 tsp. parsley and shake. In another pot, whisk the egg with a spot of table salt and pepper. Dunk chicken in egg and afterward in almond flour consolidate. Warm up a dish with 3 tbsp oil over moderate gigantic warmth, embed chicken, get ready until they are brilliant on the two sides and move to paper towels.
- In a pot, consolidate spaghetti squash with table salt, pepper, dried basil, 1 tablespoon oil and the remainder of the parsley and shake. Disperse this into a heatproof dish, embed chicken pieces and afterward the marinara sauce. Top with destroyed mozzarella, present in the broiler at 375 degrees F and prepare for 30 minutes. Embellishment new basil toward the end, leave dish aside to chill off a piece, convey among plates and serve.

Chicken Stuffed Cauliflower Florets
Ingredients:

- 2 chicken breasts, skinless, boneless, prepared and shredded
- 2 tbsp fajita seasoning
- 1 tablespoon ghee
- 2 mugs cauliflower florets
- Table salt and black pepper to the taste

- 1 small yellow onion, sliced off
- 6 bell peppers, tops slice off and seeds removed
- 2/3 mug water

Instructions:

- Put cauliflower florets in your food processor, insert a pinch of table salt and pepper, pulse well and shift to a pot. Warm up a dish with the ghee over moderate heat, insert onions, shake and prepare for 2 minutes.
- Insert cauliflower, shake and prepare for 3 minutes more. Insert seasoning, table salt, pepper, water and chicken, shake and prepare for 2 minutes. Put bell peppers on a lined baking sheet, stuff each with chicken combine, introduce in the oven at 350 degrees F and bake for 30 minutes. Distribute them between plates and serve.

Creamy Chicken
Ingredients:

- Table salt and black pepper to the taste
- ¾ mug parmesan, grated
- Preparing spray
- 8 mozzarella slices
- 4 chicken breasts, skinless and boneless
- ½ mug mayo
- ½ mug sour cream
- 1 tsp. garlic grinding grains

Instructions:

- Spray a baking dish, put chicken breasts in it and top each piece with 2 mozzarella slices. In a pot, combine pram with table salt, pepper, mayo, garlic grinding grains and sour cream and shake well. Scatter this over chicken, introduce dish in the oven at 375 degrees F and bake for 1 hour. Distribute between plates and serve.

Garlic Chicken Dish
Ingredients:

- 4 ounces cheddar cheese, cubed
- 2 ounces provolone cheese, cubed
- 1 zucchini, shredded
- 3 pounds chicken breasts
- 2 ounces muenster cheese, cubed
- 2 ounces cream cheese
- Table salt and black pepper to the taste
- 1 tsp. garlic, chopped

- ½ mug bacon, prepared and crumbled

Instructions:

- Season zucchini with table salt and pepper, leave aside few minutes, press well and shift to a pot. Insert bacon, garlic, a lot of table salt and pepper, cream cheese, cheddar cheese, muenster cheese and provolone cheese and shake.
- Slice slits into chicken breasts, season with table salt and pepper and stuff with zucchini and cheese mix. Put on a lined baking sheet, introduce within the oven at 400 degrees F and bake for forty-five minutes. Distribute between plates and serve.

Balsamic Chick

Ingredients:

- 1 mug chicken stock
- 3 tbsp stevia
- ½ mug balsamic vinegar
- 1 tomato, thinly sliced
- 3 tbsp coconut oil
- 2 pounds chicken breasts, skinless and boneless
- 3 garlic cloves, chopped
- Table salt and black pepper to the taste
- 6 mozzarella slices
- Some sliced off basil for serving

Instructions:

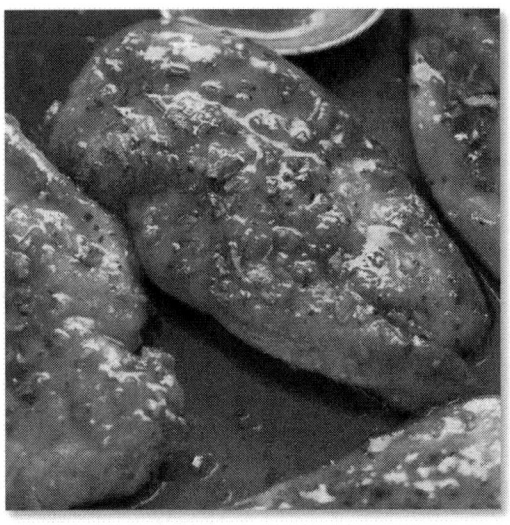

- Warm up a dish with the oil over moderate immense heat, insert chicken items, season with table salt and pepper, prepare till they brown on each side and reduce heat. Insert garlic, vinegar, stock and stevia, shake, expand heat again and prepare for ten minutes.
- Shift chicken breasts to a lined baking sheet, organize mozzarella slices on high, then prime with basil. Broil in the oven over moderate heat until cheese melts and then Organize tomato slices over chicken items. Distribute between plates and serve.

Salted Crusted Chicken

Ingredients:

- ½ mug avocado oil
- 1 egg, whisked
- Table salt and black pepper to the taste
- 1 mug asiago cheese, shredded
- 4 bacon slices, prepared and crumbled

- 4 chicken breasts, skinless and boneless
- 1 tablespoon water
- ¼ tsp. garlic grinding grains
- 1 mug parmesan cheese, grated

Instructions:

- In a pot, combine parmesan cheese with garlic, table salt and pepper and shake. Put whisked egg in another pot and combine with the water. Season chicken with table salt and pepper and dip each piece into egg and then into cheese combine.
- Warm up a dish with the oil over moderate immense heat, insert chicken breasts, prepare until they are golden on both sides and shift to a baking dish. Introduce in the oven at 350 degrees F and bake for 20 minutes. Top chicken with bacon and asiago cheese, introduce in the oven, turn on broiler and broil for a couple of minutes. Serve warm.

Peanut Grilled Chicken
Ingredients:

- A pinch of red pepper flakes
- Table salt and black pepper to the taste
- ½ tsp. ginger, ground
- 1/3 mug peanut butter
- 2 and ½ pounds chicken and drumsticks
- 1 tablespoon coconut aminos
- 1 tablespoon apple cider vinegar
- 1 garlic clove, chopped
- ½ mug warm water

Instructions:

- In your blender combine peanut butter with water, aminos, table salt, pepper, pepper flakes, ginger, garlic and vinegar and blend well. Pat dry chicken pieces organize them in a dish and pour the peanut butter marinade over it.
- Fling to coat and keep in the fridge for 1 hour. Put chicken pieces skin side down on your preheated grill over moderate immense heat, prepare for 10 minutes, flip, brush with some of the marinades and prepare them for 10 minutes more. Distribute between plates and serve.

Tomato Chicken
Ingredients:

- 2 chicken breasts, skinless and boneless and sliced
- 1 tomato, sliced off
- ½ tsp. oregano, dried
- ½ tsp. basil, dried
- 1 zucchini, sliced off
- Table salt and black pepper to the taste

- 1 tsp. garlic grinding grains
- 1 tablespoon avocado oil
- ½ mug mozzarella cheese, shredded

Instructions:

- Season chicken with table salt, pepper and garlic grinding grains. Warm up a dish with the oil over moderate heat, insert chicken slices, brown on all sides and shift them to a baking dish. Warm up the dish again over moderate heat, insert zucchini, oregano, tomato, basil, table salt and pepper, shake, prepare for two minutes and pour over chicken.
- Introduce within the oven at 325 degrees F and bake for twenty minutes. Scatter mozzarella over chicken, introduce in the oven once more and bake for five minutes more. Distribute between plates and serve.

Bacon Wrapped Chicken

Ingredients:

- 2 pounds chicken breasts, skinless and boneless
- 12 bacon slices
- 1 tablespoon chives, sliced off
- 8 ounces cream cheese
- Table salt and black pepper to the taste

Instructions:

- Warm up a dish over moderate heat, insert bacon, prepare until its 0.5 done, shift to paper towels and drain grease. In an exceedingly pot, mix cream cheese with table salt, pepper and chives and shake. Use a meat tenderizer to flatten chicken breasts well, distribute cream cheese mix, roll them up and wrap each during a prepared bacon slice.
- Organize wrapped chicken breasts into a baking dish, introduce within the oven at 375 degrees F and bake for thirty minutes. Distribute between plates and serve.

Malia Botti Chicken Wings

Ingredients:

- 3 tbsp rice vinegar
- 3 tbsp stevia
- ¼ mug scallions, sliced off
- ½ tsp. xanthan gum
- 3 pounds chicken wings
- Table salt and black pepper to the taste
- 3 tbsp coconut aminos
- 2 teaspoons white vinegar
- 5 dried chilies, sliced off

Instructions:

- Scatter chicken wings on a lined baking sheet, season with table salt and pepper, introduce within the oven at 375 degrees F and bake for forty-five minutes.
- Meanwhile, heat up a small dish over moderate heat, insert white vinegar, rice vinegar, coconut aminos, stevia, xanthan gum, scallions and chilies, shake well, bring to a boil, prepare for two minutes and take away heat. Dip chicken wings into this sauce, organize all of them on the baking sheet again and bake for ten minutes additional. Serve them heat.

Chicken Tim menses in Creamy Sauce
Ingredients:

- 4 bacon strips, sliced off
- 4 garlic cloves, chopped
- 10 ounces cremini mushrooms, halved
- 2 mugs white chardonnay wine
- 1 mug whipping cream
- 8 chicken
- Table salt and black pepper to the taste
- 1 yellow onion, sliced off
- 1 tablespoon coconut oil
- A handful parsley, sliced off

Instructions:

- Warm up a dish with the oil over moderate heat, insert bacon, shake, prepare till it's crispy, take away heat and shift to paper towels. Warm up the dish with the bacon fat over moderate heat, insert chicken pieces, season them with table salt and pepper, prepare till they brown and conjointly shift to paper towels.
- Warm up the dish again over moderate heat, insert onions, shake and prepare for six minutes. Insert garlic, shake, prepare for 1 minute and shift next to bacon items. Return dish to stove and Warm up again over moderate tempera. Insert mushrooms shake and prepare them for five minutes.
- Return chicken, bacon, garlic and onion to dish. Insert wine, shake, bring to a boil, reduce heat and simmer for 40 minutes. Insert parsley and cream, shake and prepare for ten minutes additional. Distribute between plates and serve.

Yellow Onion Chicken
Ingredients:

- 8 ounces cream cheese
- ¼ mug yellow onion, sliced off
- ½ mug mayonnaise
- ½ mug parmesan, grated
- 1 mug cheddar cheese, grated
- 6 chicken breasts, skinless and boneless

- Table salt and black pepper to the taste
- ¼ mug jalapenos, sliced off
- 5 bacon slices, sliced off
- 2 ounces pork skins, crushed
- 4 tbsp melted ghee
- ½ mug parmesan

Instructions:

Put together chicken bosoms in a preparing dish, season with table salt and pepper, present in the stove at 425 degrees F and heat for 40 minutes. Then, Warm up a dish over moderate warmth, embed bacon, shake, get ready until it's fresh and move to a plate. Warm up the dish again over moderate warmth, embed onions, shake and get ready for 4 minutes. Eliminate heat, embed bacon, jalapeno, cream cheddar, mayo, cheddar and ½ mug pram and shake well. Dissipate this over chicken. In a pot, join pork skin with ghee and ½ mug pram and shake. Disperse this over chicken too, present in the stove and heat for 15 minutes more. Serve warm.

Chicken and Sour Cream Sauce

Ingredients:

- 1 tsp. onion grinding grains
- ¼ mug sour cream
- 4 chicken
- Table salt and black pepper to the taste
- 2 tbsp sweet paprika

Instructions:

- In a pot, combine paprika with table salt, pepper and onion grinding grains and shake. Season chicken pieces with this paprika combine, organize them on a lined baking sheet and bake in the oven at 400 degrees F for 40 minutes.
- Distribute chicken on plates and leave aside for now. Pour juices from the dish into a pot and insert sour cream. Shake this sauce very well and drizzle over chicken.

Chicken Gumbo

Ingredients:

- 28 ounces canned tomatoes, sliced off
- 3 tbsp thyme, dried
- 2 tbsp garlic grinding grains
- 2 tbsp mustard grinding grains
- 1 tsp. cayenne grinding grains
- 2 sausages, sliced
- 3 chicken breasts, cubed
- 2 tbsp oregano, dried
- 2 bell peppers, sliced off

- 1 small yellow onion, sliced off
- 1 tbsp chili grinding grains
- Table salt and black pepper to the taste
- 6 tbsp Creole seasoning

Instructions:

- In your slow preparer, combine sausages with chicken pieces, table salt, pepper, bell peppers, oregano, onion, thyme, garlic grinding grains, mustard grinding grains, tomatoes, cayenne, chili and Creole seasoning.
- Wrap up and prepare on Low for 7 hours. Unwrap up pot again, shake gumbo and Distribute into pots. Serve warm.

Tender Chicken Tim menses
Ingredients:

- 2 garlic cloves, chopped
- 6 chicken, skin and bone-in
- 3 tbsp ghee
- 8 ounces mushrooms, sliced
- 2 tbsp gruyere cheese, grated
- Table salt and black pepper to the taste

Instructions:

- Warm up a dish with 1 tablespoon ghee over moderate warmth, embed chicken, season with table salt and pepper, get ready for 3 minutes on each side and Organize them in a heating dish. Warm up the dish again with the remainder of the ghee over moderate warmth, embed garlic, shake and plan for 1 moment.
- Supplement mushrooms and shake well. Addition table salt and pepper, shake and get ready for 10 minutes. Spoon these over chickens, Garnish cheddar, present in the stove at 350 degrees F and heat for 30 minutes. Go stove to oven and cook everything for a couple more minutes. Appropriate among plates and serve.

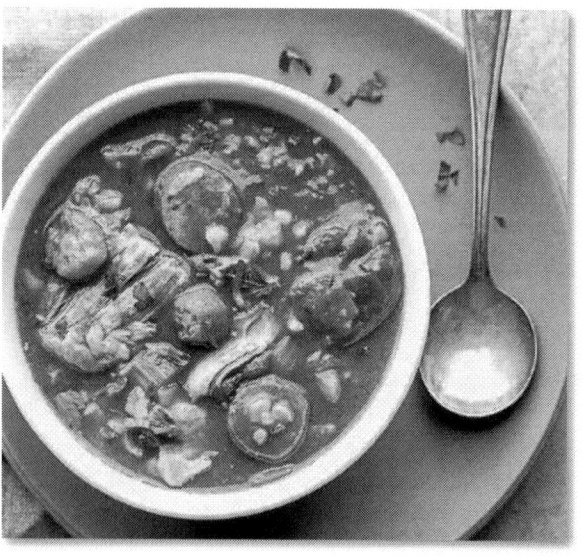

Crusted Chicken

Ingredients:

- 1 and ½ mugs pecans, sliced off
- 4 chicken breasts
- Table salt and black pepper to the taste
- 1 egg, whisked
- Table salt and black pepper to the taste
- 3 tbsp coconut oil

Instructions:

- Put pecans in a pot and the whisked egg in another. Season chicken, dip in egg and then in pecans. Warm up a dish with the oil over moderate immense heat, insert chicken and prepare until it's brown on both sides.
- Shift chicken pieces to a baking sheet, introduce in the oven and bake at 350 degrees F for 10 minutes. Distribute between plates and serve.

Pepperoni Chicken Breasts Bake

Ingredients:

- Table salt and black pepper to the taste
- 1 tsp. oregano, dried
- 6 ounces mozzarella, sliced
- 14 ounces low carb pizza sauce
- 1 tablespoon coconut oil
- 4 moderate chicken breasts, skinless and boneless
- 1 tsp. garlic grinding grains
- 2 ounces pepperoni, sliced

Instructions:

- Put pizza sauce in a very tiny pot, bring to a boil over moderate heat, simmer for 20 minutes and remove heat. During a pot, mix chicken with table salt, pepper, garlic grinding grains and oregano and shake.
- Warm up a dish with the coconut oil over moderate immense heat, insert chicken pieces, prepare for two minutes on every side and shift them to a baking dish. Insert mozzarella slices on high, Scatter sauce, prime with pepperoni slices, introduce in the oven at 400 degrees F and bake for thirty minutes. Distribute between plates and serve.

Mexican Double Chicken Soup

Ingredients:

- 15 ounces canned chunky salsa
- 8 ounces Monterey jack

- 1 and ½ pounds chicken tights, skinless, boneless and cubed
- 15 ounces chicken stock

Instructions:

- In your slow preparer, combine chicken with stock, salsa and cheese, shake, wrap up and prepare on Immense for 4 hours. Unwrap up pot, shake soup, distribute into pots and serve.

Spinach and Parmesan Chicken
Ingredients:

- 10 ounces spinach
- ½ mug parmesan, grated
- 1 tablespoon dried onion
- 1 tablespoon garlic, dried
- 4 ounces cream cheese
- 4 chicken breasts
- 10 ounces canned artichoke hearts, sliced off
- Table salt and black pepper to the taste
- 4 ounces mozzarella, shredded

Instructions:

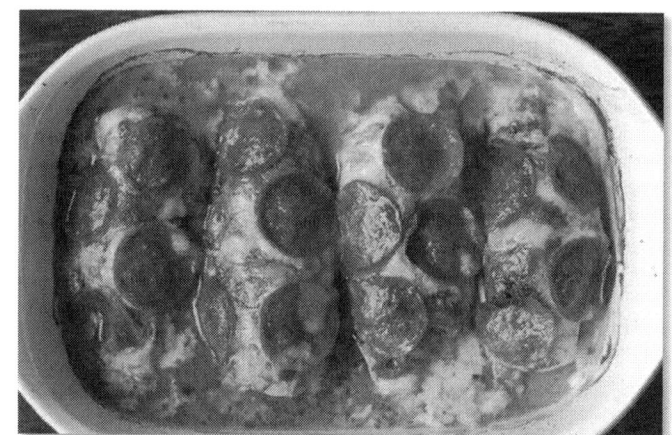

- Put chicken bosoms on a lined preparing sheet, season with table salt and pepper, present in the stove at 400 degrees F and heat for 30 minutes.
- In a pot, consolidate artichokes with onion, cream cheddar, parmesan, spinach, garlic, table salt and pepper and shake. Remove chicken from the broiler, cut each piece in the center, disseminate artichokes consolidate, Garnish mozzarella, present in the stove at 400 degrees F and prepare for 15 minutes more. Serve warm.

Chicken Meatloaf
Ingredients:

- 2 teaspoons Italian seasoning
- Table salt and black pepper to the taste
- ½ mug ricotta cheese
- 1 mug parmesan, grated
- 1 mug mozzarella, shredded
- 1 mug marinara sauce
- 2-pound chicken meat, ground

- 2 tbsp parsley, sliced off
- 4 garlic cloves, chopped
- 2 teaspoons onion grinding grains
- 2 teaspoons chives, sliced off
- 2 tbsp parsley, sliced off
- 1 garlic clove, chopped

Instructions:

- In a pot, join chicken with half of the marinara sauce, table salt, pepper, Italian flavoring, 4 garlic cloves, onion granulating grains and 2 tbsp parsley and shake well. In another pot, consolidate ricotta with half of the parmesan, half of the mozzarella, chives, 1 garlic clove, table salt, pepper and 2 tbsp parsley and shake well.
- Put half of the chicken consolidate into a portion dish and Scatter equally. Addition cheddar filling and furthermore Scatter.
- Top with the remainder of the meat and Scatter once more. Present meatloaf in the broiler at 400 degrees F and prepare for 20 minutes. Remove meatloaf from the broiler, Scatter the remainder of the marinara sauce, the remainder of the parmesan and mozzarella and heat for 20 minutes more. Leave meatloaf to chill off, cut, disseminate among plates and serve.

Whole Chicken

Ingredients:

- Table salt and black pepper to the taste
- 2 tbsp coconut oil
- 1 tsp. Italian seasoning
- 1 and ½ mugs chicken stock
- 1 whole chicken
- ½ tsp. onion grinding grains
- ½ tsp. garlic grinding grains
- 2 teaspoons guar parsley, sliced

Instructions:

- Rub chicken with 0.5 of the oil, garlic grinding grains, table salt, pepper, Italian seasoning and onion grinding grains. Put the remainder of the oil into an immediate pot and insert chicken to the pot.
- Insert stock, conclude pot and prepare on Immense for 40 minutes. Shift chicken to a platter and leave aside for now. Set the moment pot on Sauté mode, insert guar parsley, sliced, shake and prepare until it thickens. Pour sauce over chicken and serve.

Chicken and Green Onion Sauce

Ingredients:

4 chicken breast halves, skinless and boneless

- Table salt and black pepper to the taste
- 2 tbsp ghee
- 1 green onion, sliced off
- 8 ounces sour cream

Instructions:

- Warm up a dish with the ghee over moderate immense heat, insert chicken items, season with table salt and pepper, wrap up, reduce heat and simmer for ten minutes. Unwrap up dish, turn chicken items and prepare them Wrap upped for ten minutes additional.
- Insert inexperienced onions, shake and prepare for 2 minutes a lot of. Remove heat, insert additional table salt and pepper if required, insert sour cream, shake well, wrap up dish and leave aside for 5 minutes. Shake once more, distribute between plates and serve.

Chicken Creamy Stuffed Mushrooms

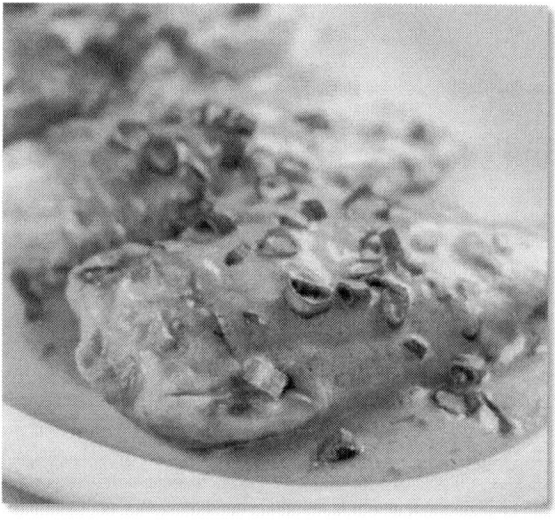

Ingredients:

- ¾ mug blue cheese, crumbled
- ¼ mug red onion, sliced off
- ½ mug chicken meat, already prepared and sliced off
- Table salt and black pepper to the taste
- 16 ounces button mushroom caps
- 4 ounces cream cheese
- ¼ mug carrot, sliced off
- 1 tsp. ranch seasoning combine
- 4 tbsp warm sauce
- Preparing spray

Instructions:

- In a pot, combine cream cheese with blue cheese, warm sauce, ranch seasoning, table salt, pepper, chicken, carrot and red onion and shake.
- Stuff each mushroom cap with this combine, put them all on a lined baking sheet, spray with preparing spray, introduce in the oven at 425 degrees F and bake for 10 minutes. Distribute between plates and serve them.

Chicken Onion Stroganoff

Ingredients:

- 1 mug coconut milk
- 1 yellow onion, sliced off
- 1-pound chicken breasts, slice into moderate pieces
- 1 and ½ teaspoons thyme, dried
- 2 tbsp parsley, sliced off
- 2 garlic cloves, chopped
- 8 ounces mushrooms, roughly sliced off
- ¼ tsp. celery seeds, ground
- 1 mug chicken stock
- Table salt and black pepper to the teste
- 4 zucchinis, slice with a spiralizer

Instructions:

- Put chicken in your slow preparer. Insert table salt, pepper, onion, garlic, mushrooms, coconut milk, celery seeds, stock, 0.5 of the parsley and thyme. Shake, finish off and prepare on Immense for four hours.
- Unwrap up pot, insert a lot of table salt and pepper if required and the rest of the parsley and shake. Warm up a dish with water over moderate heat, insert some table salt, bring to a boil, insert zucchini pasta, prepare for one minute and drain. Distribute on plates, insert chicken combine on prime and serve.

Lemon Herb Chicken

Ingredients:

- 12 ounces boneless, skinless chicken breast, cut into 8 strips
- 1 small egg white
- 2 tablespoons water, divided
- ½ cup breadcrumbs
- ¼ cup unsalted butter, divided
- Juice of 1 lemon
- Zest of 1 lemon
- 1 tablespoon fresh chopped basil
- 1 teaspoon fresh chopped thyme
- Lemon slices, for garnish

Instructions:

- Place the chicken strips between 2 sheets of plastic wrap and pound each flat with a mallet or rolling pin.
- In a medium bowl, whisk together the egg and 1 tablespoon water.
- Put the breadcrumbs in another medium bowl.
- Dredge the chicken strips, one at a time, in the egg, then the breadcrumbs, and set the breaded strips aside on a plate.
- In a large skillet over medium heat, melt 2 tablespoons of the butter.

- Cook the strips in the butter for about 3 minutes, turning once, or until they are golden and cooked through.
- Transfer the chicken to a plate.
- Add the lemon juice, lemon zest, basil, thyme, and remaining 1 tablespoon water to the skillet and stir until the mixture simmers.
- Remove the sauce from the heat and stir in the remaining 2 tablespoons butter.
- Serve the chicken with the lemon sauce drizzled over the top and garnished with lemon slices.

Asian Chicken Satay

Ingredients:

- Juice of 2 limes
- 2 tablespoons brown sugar
- 1 tablespoon minced garlic
- 2 teaspoons ground cumin
- 12 ounces boneless, skinless chicken breast, cut into 12 strips

Instructions:

- In a large bowl, stir together the lime juice, brown sugar, garlic, and cumin.
- Add the chicken strips to the bowl and marinate in the refrigerator for 1 hour.
- Heat the barbecue to medium-high.
- Remove the chicken from the marinade and thread each strip onto wooden skewers that have been soaked in water.
- Grill the chicken for about 4 minutes per side or until the meat is cooked through but still juicy.

Indian Chicken Curry

Ingredients:

- 3 tablespoons olive oil, divided
- 6 boneless, skinless chicken thighs
- 1 small, sweet onion
- 2 teaspoons minced garlic
- 1 teaspoon grated fresh ginger
- 1 tablespoon Hot Curry Powder (here)
- ¾ cup water
- ¼ cup coconut milk
- 2 tablespoons chopped fresh cilantro

Instructions:

- In a large skillet over a medium-high heat, heat 2 tablespoons of the oil.
- Add the chicken and cook for about 10 minutes or until the thighs are
- browned all over.
- With tongs, remove the chicken to a plate and set aside.
- Add the remaining 1 tablespoon of oil to the skillet and sauté the onion, garlic, and ginger for about 3 minutes or until they are softened.
- Stir in the curry powder, water, and coconut milk.
- Return the chicken to the skillet and bring the liquid to a boil.

- Reduce the heat to low, cover the skillet, and simmer for about 25 minutes or until the chicken is tender and the sauce is thick.
- Serve topped with cilantro.

Persian Chicken

Ingredients:

- ½ small, sweet onion, chopped
- ¼ cup freshly squeezed lemon juice
- 1 tablespoon dried oregano
- 1 teaspoon minced garlic
- 1 teaspoon sweet paprika
- ½ teaspoon ground cumin
- ½ cup olive oil
- 5 boneless, skinless chicken thighs

Instructions:

- Put the onion, lemon juice, oregano, garlic, paprika, and cumin in a blender or food processor.
- Pulse a few times to mix the ingredients.
- With the motor running, add the olive oil until the mixture is smooth.
- Place the chicken thighs in a large sealable freezer bag and pour the marinade into the bag.
- Seal the bag and place it in the refrigerator, turning the bag twice, for 2 hours.
- Remove the thighs from the marinade and discard the extra marinade.
- Preheat the barbecue to medium.
- Grill the chicken for about 20 minutes, turning once, or until the internal temperature is 165°F.

Pesto Pork Chops

Ingredients:

- 4 (3-ounce) pork top-loin chops, boneless, fat trimmed
- 8 teaspoons Herb Pesto (here)
- ½ cup breadcrumbs
- 1 tablespoon olive oil

Instructions:

- Preheat the oven to 450°F.
- Line a baking sheet with foil; set aside.
- Rub 1 teaspoon of pesto evenly over both sides of each pork chop.
- Lightly dredge each pork chop in the breadcrumbs.
- In a large skillet over medium-high heat, heat the oil.
- Brown the pork chops on each side for about 5 minutes.
- Place the pork chops on the baking sheet.
- Bake for about 10 minutes or until the pork reaches 145°F in the center.

Pork Souvlaki

Ingredients:

- 3 tablespoons olive oil
- 2 tablespoons lemon juice
- 1 teaspoon minced garlic
- 1 tablespoon chopped fresh oregano
- ¼ teaspoon freshly ground black pepper
- 1-pound pork leg, cut in 2-inch cubes

Instructions:

- In a medium bowl, stir together the olive oil, lemon juice, garlic, oregano,
- and pepper.
- Add the pork cubes and toss to coat.
- Place the bowl in the refrigerator, covered, for 2 hours to marinate.
- Thread the pork chunks onto 8 metal skewers or wood skewers that have
- been soaked in water.
- Preheat the barbecue to medium-high heat.
- Grill the pork skewers for about 12 minutes, turning once, until just cooked
- through but still juicy.

Chili Roasted Pork Leg

Ingredients:

- 2 teaspoons chili powder
- 2 teaspoons ground allspice
- 1½ teaspoons ground cumin
- 1 teaspoon garlic powder
- 1 teaspoon ground cinnamon
- ½ teaspoon freshly ground black pepper
- Pinch cayenne pepper
- 1-pound boneless pork leg roast
- 2 tablespoons olive oil

Instructions:

- In a small bowl, mix together the chili powder, allspice, cumin, garlic powder, cinnamon, black pepper, and cayenne pepper.
- Rub the spice mixture generously all over the pork leg.
- Place the pork loin in the refrigerator to marinate for 3 hours.
- Preheat the oven to 350°F.
- In a large skillet over medium-high heat, heat the olive oil.
- Sear the pork loin on all sides and transfer it to a baking dish.
- Roast, uncovered, for about 40 minutes or until the internal temperature reaches 160°F.
- Remove the pork from the oven and let it rest for 10 minutes.
- Cut into thin slices to serve.

Open Faced Beef Stir Up

Ingredients:

- ½ pound 95% lean ground beef
- ½ cup chopped sweet onion
- ½ cup shredded cabbage
- ¼ cup Herb Pesto (here)
- 6 hamburger buns, bottom halves only

Instructions:

- In a large skillet over medium heat, sauté the beef and onion for about 6 minutes or until the beef is cooked.
- Add the cabbage and sauté for 3 additional minutes.
- Stir in the pesto and heat for 1 minute.
- Divide the beef mixture into 6 portions and serve each on the bottom half of a hamburger bun, open face.

Sweet and Sour Meat Loaf

Ingredients:

- 1 pound 95% lean ground beef
- ½ cup breadcrumbs
- ½ cup chopped sweet onion
- 1 large egg
- 2 tablespoons chopped fresh basil
- 1 teaspoon chopped fresh thyme
- 1 teaspoon chopped fresh parsley
- ¼ teaspoon freshly ground black pepper
- 1 tablespoon brown sugar
- 1 teaspoon white vinegar
- ¼ teaspoon garlic powder

Instructions:

- Preheat the oven to 350°F.
- Mix together the beef, breadcrumbs, onion, egg, basil, thyme, parsley, and pepper until well combined.
- Press the meat mixture into a 9-by-5-inch loaf pan.
- In a small bowl, stir together the brown sugar, vinegar, and garlic powder.
- Spread the brown sugar mixture evenly over the meat.
- Bake the meat loaf for about 50 minutes or until it is cooked through.
- Let the meat loaf stand for 10 minutes and then pour out any accumulated grease.

Grilled Steak with Cucumber Cilantro Salsa

Ingredients:

FOR THE SALSA

- 1 cup chopped English cucumber
- ¼ cup boiled and diced red bell pepper
- 1 scallion, both green and white parts, chopped
- 2 tablespoons chopped fresh cilantro
- Juice of 1 lime

FOR THE STEAK

- 4 (3-ounce) beef tenderloin steaks
- Olive oil
- Freshly ground black pepper

Instructions:

TO MAKE THE SALSA

- In a medium bowl, combine the cucumber, bell pepper, scallion, cilantro, and lime juice; set aside.

TO MAKE THE STEAK

- Preheat a barbecue to medium-high.
- Take the steaks out of the refrigerator and let them come to room temperature.
- Rub the steaks all over with olive oil and season with pepper.
- Grill the steaks for about 5 minutes per side for medium-rare, or until desired doneness.
- If you do not have a barbecue, broil the steaks in the oven for 6 minutes per side for medium-rare.
- Let the steaks rest for 10 minutes.
- Serve the steaks topped with the salsa.

Classic Pot Roast

Ingredients:

- 1-pound boneless beef chuck or rump roast
- ½ teaspoon freshly ground black pepper
- 1 tablespoon olive oil
- ½ small, sweet onion, chopped
- 2 teaspoons minced garlic
- 1 teaspoon dried thyme
- 1 cup plus 3 tablespoons water
- 2 tablespoons cornstarch

Instructions:

- Place a large stockpot over medium heat.
- Season the roast with pepper.
- Add the oil to the stockpot and brown the meat all over.
- Remove the meat to a plate; set aside.

- Sauté the onion and garlic in the stockpot for about 3 minutes or until they are softened.
- Return the beef to the pot with any accumulated juices and add the thyme and 1 cup water.
- Bring the liquid to a boil and then reduce the heat to low so that the liquid
- simmers.
- Cover and simmer for about 4½ hours or until the beef is very tender.
- In a small bowl, stir together the cornstarch and 3 tablespoons water to form a slurry.
- Whisk the slurry into the liquid in the pot and cook for 15 minutes to thicken the sauce.
- Serve the roast with the gravy.

Grilled Calamari with Lemon and Herbs

Ingredients:

- 2 tablespoons olive oil
- 2 tablespoons freshly squeezed lemon juice
- 1 tablespoon chopped fresh parsley
- 1 tablespoon chopped fresh oregano
- 2 teaspoons minced garlic
- Pinch sea salt
- Pinch freshly ground black pepper
- ½ pound cleaned calamari
- Lemon wedges, for garnish

Instructions:

- In large bowl, stir together the olive oil, lemon juice, parsley, oregano, garlic, salt, and pepper.
- Add the calamari to the bowl and stir to coat.
- Cover the bowl and refrigerate the calamari for 1 hour to marinate.
- Preheat the barbecue to medium-high.
- Grill the calamari, turning once, until firm and opaque, about 3 minutes total.
- Serve with lemon wedges

Herbs Pesto Tuna

Ingredients:

- 4 (3-ounce) yellowfin tuna fillets
- 1 teaspoon olive oil
- Freshly ground black pepper
- ¼ cup Herb Pesto (see here)
- 1 lemon, cut into 8 thin slices

Instructions:

- Heat the barbecue to medium-high.
- Drizzle the fish with the olive oil and season each fillet with pepper.
- Cook the fish on the barbecue for 4 minutes.
- Turn the fish over and top each piece with the herb pesto and lemon slices.
- Grill for 5 to 6 minutes more or until the tuna is cooked too medium-well.

Cilantro Lime Flounder

Ingredients:

- ¼ cup Homemade Mayonnaise (here)
- Juice of 1 lime
- Zest of 1 lime
- ½ cup chopped fresh cilantro
- 4 (3-ounce) flounder fillets
- Freshly ground black pepper

Instructions:

- Preheat the oven to 400°F.
- In a small bowl, stir together the mayonnaise, lime juice, lime zest, and cilantro.
- Place 4 pieces of foil, about 8 by 8 inches square, on a clean work surface.
- Place a flounder fillet in the center of each square.
- Top the fillets evenly with the mayonnaise mixture.
- Season the flounder with pepper.
- Fold the sides of the foil over the fish, creating a snug packet, and place the
- foil packets on a baking sheet.
- Bake the fish 4 to 5 minutes.
- Unfold the packets and serve.

Shore Lunch Style Sole

Ingredients:

- ¼ cup all-purpose flour
- ¼ teaspoon freshly ground black pepper
- 12 ounces sole fillets, deboned and skinned
- 2 tablespoons olive oil
- 1 scallion, both green and white parts, chopped
- Lemon wedges, for garnish

Instructions:

- In a large plastic freezer bag, shake together the flour and pepper to combine.
- Add the fish fillets to the flour and shake to coat.
- In a large skillet over medium-high heat, heat the olive oil.
- When the oil is hot, add the fish fillets and fry for about 10 minutes, turning once, or until they are golden and cooked through.
- Remove the fish from the oil onto paper towels to drain.
- Serve topped with chopped scallions and a squeeze of lemon.

Herb Crusted Baker Haddock

Ingredients:

- ½ cup breadcrumbs
- 3 tablespoons chopped fresh parsley
- 1 tablespoon lemon zest
- 1 teaspoon chopped fresh thyme
- ¼ teaspoon freshly ground black pepper

- 1 tablespoon melted unsalted butter
- 12-ounces haddock fillets, deboned and skinned

Instructions:

- Preheat the oven to 350°F.
- In a small bowl, stir together the breadcrumbs, parsley, lemon zest, thyme, and pepper until well combined.
- Add the melted butter and toss until the mixture resembles coarse crumbs.
- Place the haddock on a baking sheet and spoon the bread crumb mixture on top, pressing down firmly.
- Bake the haddock in the oven for about 20 minutes or until the fish is just
- cooked through and flakes off in chunks when pressed.

Roasted Beef Stew

Ingredients:

- ¼ cup all-purpose flour
- 1 teaspoon freshly ground black pepper, plus extra for seasoning
- Pinch cayenne pepper
- ½ pound boneless beef chuck roast, trimmed of fat and cut into 1-inch chunks
- 2 tablespoons olive oil
- ½ sweet onion, chopped
- 2 teaspoons minced garlic
- 1 cup homemade beef stock
- 1 cup plus 2 tablespoons water
- 1 carrot, cut into ½-inch chunks
- 2 celery stalks, chopped with greens
- 1 teaspoon chopped fresh thyme
- 1 teaspoon cornstarch
- 2 tablespoons chopped fresh parsley

Instructions:

- Preheat the oven to 350°F.
- Put the flour, black pepper, and cayenne pepper in a large plastic freezer bag and toss to mix.
- Add the beef chunks to the bag and toss to coat.
- In a large ovenproof pot, heat the olive oil.
- Sauté the beef chunks for about 5 minutes or until they are lightly browned.
- Remove the beef from the pot and set aside on a plate.
- Add the onion and garlic to the pot and sauté for 3 minutes.
- Stir in the beef stock and deglaze the pot, scraping up any bits on the bottom.
- Add 1 cup water, the beef drippings on the plate, the carrot, celery, and thyme.
- Cover the pot tightly with a lid or aluminum foil and place in the oven.
- Bake the stew, stirring occasionally, for about 1 hour or until the meat is very tender.
- Remove the stew from the oven.
- In a small bowl, stir together the 2 tablespoons water and the cornstarch and then stir the mixture into the hot stew to thicken the sauce.
- Season the stew with black pepper and serve topped with parsley.

Ground Beef and Rice Soup

Ingredients:

- ½ pound extra-lean ground beef
- ½ small, sweet onion, chopped
- 1 teaspoon minced garlic
- 2 cups water
- 1 cup homemade low-sodium beef broth
- ½ cup long-grain white rice, uncooked
- 1 celery stalk, chopped
- ½ cup fresh green beans, cut into 1-inch pieces
- 1 teaspoon chopped fresh thyme
- Freshly ground black pepper

Instructions:

- Place a large saucepan over medium-high heat and add the ground beef.
- Sauté, stirring often, for about 6 minutes or until the beef is completely browned.
- Drain off the excess fat and add the onion and garlic to the saucepan.
- Sauté the vegetables for about 3 minutes or until they are softened.
- Add the water, beef broth, rice, and celery.
- Bring the soup to a boil, reduce the heat to low, and simmer for about 30 minutes or until the rice is tender.
- Add the green beans and thyme and simmer for 3 minutes.
- Remove the soup from the heat and season with pepper.

Turkey Bulgur Soup

Ingredients:

- 1 teaspoon olive oil
- ½ pound cooked ground turkey, 93% lean
- ½ sweet onion, chopped
- 1 teaspoon minced garlic
- 4 cups water
- 1 cup Easy Chicken Stock (here)
- 1 celery stalk, chopped
- 1 carrot, sliced thin
- ½ cup shredded green cabbage
- ½ cup bulgur
- 2 dried bay leaves
- 2 tablespoons chopped fresh parsley
- 1 teaspoon chopped fresh sage
- 1 teaspoon chopped fresh thyme
- Pinch red pepper flakes
- Freshly ground black pepper

Instructions:

- Place a large saucepan over medium-high heat and add the olive oil. Sauté the turkey for about 5 minutes or until the meat is cooked through.

- Add the onion and garlic and sauté for about 3 minutes or until the vegetables are softened. Add the water, chicken stock, celery, carrot, cabbage, bulgur, and bay leaves.
- Bring the soup to a boil and then reduce the heat to low and simmer for about 35 minutes or until the bulgur and vegetables are tender.
- Remove the bay leaves and stir in the parsley, sage, thyme, and red pepper flakes.
- Season with pepper and serve.

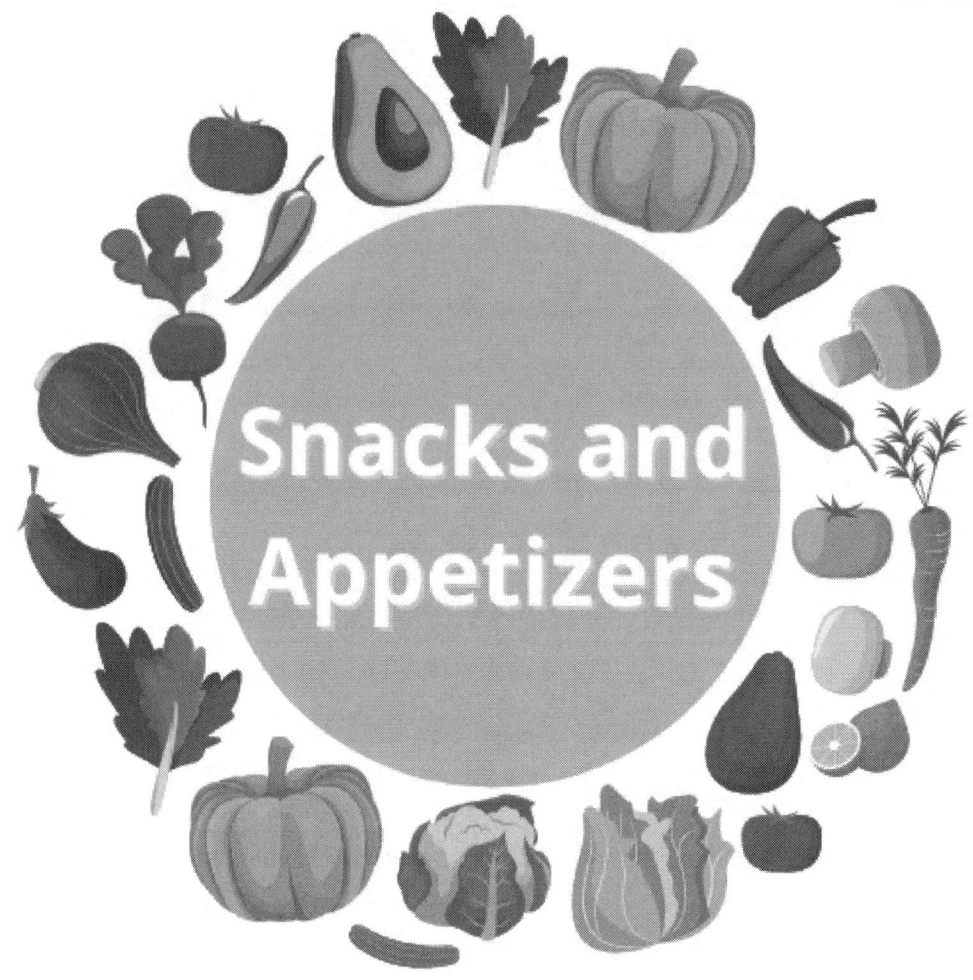

Chapter 5: Snacks and Appetizers Recipes

Onion and Cauliflower Dip

Ingredients:

- ½ mug yellow onion, sliced off
- ¾ mug cream cheese
- ½ tsp. chili grinding grains
- ½ tsp. cumin, ground
- 1 and ½ mugs chicken stock
- 1 cauliflower head, florets separated
- ¼ mug mayonnaise
- ½ tsp. garlic grinding grains
- Table salt and black pepper to the taste

Instructions:

- Put the stock in an exceedingly pot, insert cauliflower and onion, Warm up over moderate heat and prepare for 30 minutes. Insert chili grinding grains, table salt, pepper, cumin and garlic grinding grains and shake.
- Also insert cream cheese and shake a bit till it melts. Blend using an immersion blender and combine with the mayo. Shift to a pot and keep in the fridge for two hours before you serve it.

Basil Pesto Crackers
Ingredients:

- ¼ tsp. basil, dried
- 1 garlic clove, chopped
- 2 tbsp basil pesto
- A pinch of cayenne pepper
- ½ tsp. baking grinding grains
- Table salt and black pepper to the taste
- 1 and ¼ mugs almond flour
- 3 tbsp ghee

Instructions:

- In a pot, combine table salt, pepper, baking grinding grains and almond flour. Insert garlic, cayenne and basil and shake. Insert pesto and whisk. Also insert ghee and combine your dough with your finger.
- Scatter this dough on a lined baking sheet, introduce within the oven at 325 degrees F and bake for 17 minutes. Leave aside to cool down, slice your crackers and serve them as a snack.

Pumpkin Muffins
Ingredients:

- ½ mug erythritol
- ½ tsp. nutmeg, ground
- 1 tsp. cinnamon, ground
- ½ tsp. baking soda
- 1 egg
- ¼ mug sunflower seed butter
- ¾ mug pumpkin puree
- 2 tbsp flaxseed meal
- ¼ mug coconut flour
- ½ tsp. baking grinding grains
- A pinch of table salt

Instructions:

- In a pot, combine butter with pumpkin puree and egg and blend well. Insert flaxseed meal, coconut flour, erythritol, baking soda, baking grinding grains, nutmeg, cinnamon and a pinch of table salt and shake well.
- Spoon this into a greased muffin dish, introduce in the oven at 350 degrees F and bake for fifteen minutes. Leave muffins to cool down and serve them as a snack.

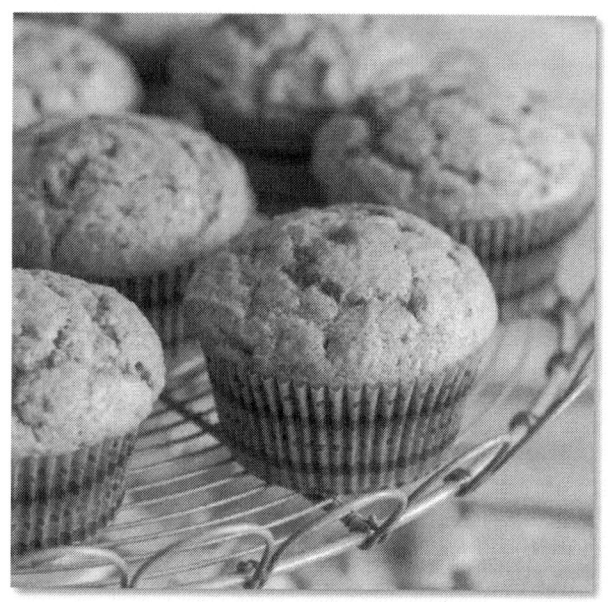

Black Pepper Bombs
Ingredients:

- 14 pepperoni slices, sliced off
- 4 ounces cream cheese
- 1 tbsp basil, sliced off
- 8 black olives, pitted and sliced off
- Table salt and black pepper to the taste
- 2 tbsp sun-dried tomato pesto

Instructions:

- In a pot, combine cream cheese with table salt, pepper, pepperoni, basil, sun dried tomato pesto and black olives and shake well. Shape balls from this combine, organize on a platter and serve.

Bacon Jalapeno Balls
Ingredients:

- 1 jalapeno pepper, sliced off
- ½ tsp. parsley, dried
- ¼ tsp. garlic grinding grains
- 3 bacon slices
- 3 ounces cream cheese
- ¼ tsp. onion grinding grains
- Table salt and black pepper to the taste

Instructions:

- Warm up a dish over moderate immense heat, insert bacon, prepare until it's crispy, shift to paper towels, drain grease and crumble. Reserve bacon fat from the dish.
- In a pot, mix cream cheese with jalapeno pepper, onion and garlic grinding grains, parsley, table salt and pepper and shake well. Insert bacon fat and bacon crumbles, shake gently, kind balls from this combine and serve.

Green Bell Peppers Pizza Dip

Ingredients:

- 1/2 mug tomato sauce
- ¼ mug mayonnaise
- ¼ mug parmesan cheese, grated
- 1 tablespoon green bell pepper, sliced off
- 6 pepperoni slices, sliced off
- 4 ounces cream cheese, soft
- ½ mug mozzarella cheese
- ¼ mug sour cream
- Table salt and black pepper to the taste
- ½ tsp. Italian seasoning
- 4 black olives, pitted and sliced off

Instructions:

- In a pot, combine cream cheese with mozzarella, bitter cream, mayo, table salt and pepper and shake well. Scatter this into 4 ramekins, insert a layer of tomato sauce, then layer parmesan cheese, top with bell pepper, pepperoni, Italian seasoning and black olives. Introduce in the oven at 350 degrees F and bake for twenty minutes. Serve warm.

Muffins Snack

Ingredients:

- A pinch of table salt
- Preparing spray
- ¼ tsp. baking grinding grains
- 1 egg
- ¼ mug coconut milk
- 1/3 mug sour cream
- ½ mug flaxseed meal
- ½ mug almond flour
- 3 tbsp swerve
- 1 tablespoon psyllium grinding grains
- 3 warm dogs, slice into 20 pieces

Instructions:

- In a pot, combine flaxseed meal with flour, psyllium grinding grains, swerve, table salt and baking grinding grains and shake. Insert egg, sour cream and coconut milk and whisk well.
- Grease a muffin tray with preparing oil, Distribute the batter you've simply build, stick a warm dog piece in the center of every muffin, introduce in the oven at 350 degrees F and bake for 12 minutes. Broil in preheated broil for 3 minutes insertional, distribute on a platter and serve.

Garlic Cloves Marinated Eggs

Ingredients:

- 2 tbsp coconut aminos
- Table salt and black pepper to the taste
- 2 garlic cloves, chopped
- 1 tsp. stevia
- 6 eggs
- 1 and ¼ mugs water
- ¼ mug unsweetened rice vinegar
- 4 ounces cream cheese
- 1 tablespoon chives, sliced off ss
-

Instructions:

- Put the eggs in an extremely pot, embed water to Wrap up, heat to the point of boiling over moderate warmth, wrap up and plan for seven minutes. Flush eggs with cold water and leave them aside to chill off wrap. In a really pot, consolidate 1 mug water with coconut aminos, vinegar, stevia and garlic and whisk well.
- Put the eggs during this join, wrap up with a kitchen towel and leave them aside for 2 hours turning at times. Strip eggs cut in equal parts and put egg yolks in a very pot. Supplement ¼ mug water, cream cheddar, table salt, pepper and chives and shake well. Stuff egg whites with this consolidate and serve them.

Bacon Crab Dip

Ingredients:

- ½ mug sour cream
- 8 ounces cream cheese
- 4 garlic cloves, chopped
- 4 green onions, chopped
- ½ mug parmesan cheese+ ½ mug parmesan cheese, grated
- Table salt and black pepper to the taste
- 2 poblano pepper, sliced off
- 8 bacon strips, sliced
- 12 ounces crab meat
- ½ mug mayonnaise
- 2 tbsp lemon juice
- Table salt and black pepper to the taste

Instructions:

- Heat up a dish over moderate immense heat, insert bacon, prepare till it's crispy, shift to paper towels, chop and leave aside to cool down. In a pot, mix butter cream with cream cheese and mayo and shake well. Insert ½ mug parmesan, poblano peppers, bacon, inexperienced onion, garlic and lemon juice and shake again.
- Insert crab meat, table salt and pepper and shake gently. Pour this into a heatproof baking dish, Scatter the rest of the pram, introduce within the oven and bake at 350 degrees F for twenty minutes. Serve your dip heat with cucumber stick.

Chia Seeds Snack

Ingredients:

- ¼ tsp. xanthan gum
- 2 tbsp olive oil
- Table salt and black pepper to the taste
- ¼ tsp. sweet paprika
- 2 tbsp psyllium husk grinding grains
- ¼ tsp. oregano, dried
- 1 and ¼ mug ice water
- ½ mug chia seeds, ground
- 3 ounces cheddar, cheese, grated
- ¼ tsp. garlic grinding grains
- ¼ tsp. onion grinding grains

Instructions:

- In a pot, combine chia seeds with xanthan gum, psyllium grinding grains, oregano, garlic and onion grinding grains, paprika, table salt and pepper and shake. Insert oil and shake well. Insert ice water and shake until you obtain a firm dough.
- Scatter this on a baking sheet, introduce within the oven at 350 degrees F and bake for 35 minutes. Leave aside to cool down, slice into 36 crackers and serve them as a snack.

Avocado Cilantro Dip

Ingredients:

- ¼ tsp. stevia
- ½ mug cilantro, sliced off
- Juice and zest of 2 limes
- ¼ mug erythritol grinding grains
- 2 avocados, pitted, peeled and slice into slices
- 1 mug coconut milk

Instructions:

- Put avocado slices on a lined baking sheet, press half of the lime juice over them and keep in your freezer for 3 hours. Warm up the coconut milk in a dish over moderate heat. Insert lime zest, shake and bring to a boil.
- Insert erythritol grinding grains, shake, remove heat and leave aside to cool down a bit. Shift avocado to your food processor, insert the rest of the lime juice and the cilantro and pulse well. Insert coconut milk combine and stevia and blend well. Shift to a pot and serve right away.

Broccoli and Cheddar Biscuits

Ingredients:

- Table salt and black pepper to the taste
- 2 eggs
- ¼ mug coconut oil
- 2 mugs cheddar cheese, grated
- 4 mugs broccoli florets
- 1 and ½ mug almond flour
- 1 tsp. paprika
- 1 tsp. garlic grinding grains
- ½ tsp. apple cider vinegar
- ½ tsp. baking soda

Instructions:

- Put broccoli florets in your food processor, insert some table salt and pepper and blend well. In a pot, combine almond flour with table salt, pepper, paprika, garlic grinding grains and baking soda and shake.
- Insert cheddar cheese, coconut oil, eggs and vinegar and shake everything. Insert broccoli and shake again. Shape 12 patties, organize on a baking sheet, introduce in the oven at 375 degrees F and bake for 20 minutes. Turn the oven to broiler and broil your biscuits for 5 minutes more. Organize on a platter and serve.

Bell Pepper Nachos

Ingredients:

- ½ tsp. oregano, dried
- ¼ tsp. red pepper flakes
- ½ mug tomato, sliced off
- Sour cream for serving
- 1-pound beef meat, ground
- 1 and ½ mugs cheddar cheese, shredded
- 1-pound mini bell peppers, slice in halves
- Table salt and black pepper to the taste
- 1 tsp. garlic grinding grains

- 1 tsp. sweet paprika
- 1 tbsp chili grinding grains
- 1 tsp. cumin, ground

Instructions:

- In a pot, mix chili grinding grains with paprika, table salt, pepper, cumin, oregano, pepper flakes and garlic grinding grains and shake.
- Warm up a dish over moderate heat, insert beef, shake and brown for ten minutes. Insert chili grinding grains combine, shake and remove heat. Organize pepper halves on a lined baking sheet, stuff them with the meat combine, Garnish cheese, introduce in the oven at four hundred degrees F and bake for ten minutes.
- Take peppers out of the oven, Garnish tomatoes and Distribute between plates and serve with bitter cream on prime.

Zucchini Snack
Ingredients:

- Table salt and black pepper to the taste
- A pinch of cumin
- 1 mug mozzarella, shredded
- ¼ mug tomato sauce
- 1 zucchini, sliced
- Preparing spray

Instructions:

- Spray a preparing sheet with some oil and Organize zucchini slices. Scatter tomato sauce all over zucchini slices, season with table salt, pepper and cumin and Garnish shredded mozzarella.
- Introduce in the oven at 350 degrees F and bake for 15 minutes. Organize on a platter and serve.

Prosciutto Appetizer
Ingredients:

- 2 tbsp erythritol
- 1/3 mug blackberries, ground
- 11 prosciuttos sliced
- 2 tbsp olive oil
- 10 ounces already prepared shrimp, peeled and deveined
- 1 tbsp mint, sliced off
- 1/3 mug red wine

Instructions:

- Wrap each shrimp in prosciutto slices, organize on a lined baking sheet, drizzle the olive oil over them, introduce in the oven at 425 degrees F and bake for 15 minutes. Warm up a dish with ground blackberries over moderate heat, insert mint, wine and erythritol, shake, prepare for 3 minutes and remove heat.
- Organize shrimp on a platter, drizzle blackberries sauce over them and serve.

Zucchini Chips

Ingredients:

- 2 tbsp olive oil
- 3 zucchinis, very thinly sliced
- Table salt and black pepper to the taste
- 2 tbsp balsamic vinegar

Instructions:

- In a pot, combine oil with vinegar, table salt and pepper and whisk well. Insert zucchini slices, fling to coat well and Scatter on a lined baking sheet, introduce in the oven at 200 degrees F and bake for 3 hours. Leave chips to cool down and serve them as a snack.

Lemon Hummus

Ingredients:

- 4 garlic cloves, chopped
- ¾ mug tahini
- ½ mug lemon juice
- 4 mugs zucchinis, finely sliced off
- ¼ mug olive oil
- Table salt and black pepper to the taste
- 1 tablespoon cumin, ground

Instructions:

- In your blender, combine zucchinis with table salt, pepper, oil, lemon juice, garlic, tahini and cumin and blend very well. Shift to a pot and serve.

Mayonnaise Celery Sticks

Ingredients:

- ¼ mug mayonnaise
- Table salt and black pepper to the taste
- ½ tsp. garlic grinding grains
- 2 mugs rotisserie chicken, shredded
- 6 celery sticks slice in halves

- 3 tbsp warm tomato sauce
- Some sliced off chives for serving

Instructions:

- In a pot, combine chicken with table salt, pepper, garlic grinding grains, mayo and tomato sauce and shake well. Organize celery pieces on a platter, Scatter chicken combine over them, garnish some chives and serve.

Beef Soya Snack
Ingredients:

- 2 tbsp black peppercorns
- 2 tbsp black pepper
- 2 pounds beef round, sliced
- 24 ounces amber
- 2 mugs soy sauce
- ½ mug Worcestershire sauce

Instructions:

- In a pot, combine soy sauce with black peppercorns, black pepper and Worcestershire sauce and whisk well. Insert beef slices, fling to coat and leave aside in the fridge for 6 hours.
- Scatter this on a rack, introduce in the oven at 370 degrees F and bake for 4 hours. Shift to a pot and serve.

Chicken Egg Roll
Ingredients:

- 2 celery stalks, finely sliced off
- ½ mug tomato sauce
- ½ tsp. erythritol
- 12 egg roll wrappers
- 4 ounces blue cheese
- 2 mugs chicken, prepared and finely sliced off
- Table salt and black pepper to the taste
- 2 green onions, sliced off
- Vegetable oil

Instructions:

In a pot, combine chicken meat with blue cheese, table salt, pepper, inexperienced onions, celery, tomato sauce and sweetener, shake well and keep within the fridge for 2 hours. Put egg wrappers on a working surface, distribute chicken combine on them, roll and seal edges. Warm up a dish with vegetable oil over moderate immense heat, insert egg rolls, prepare till they're golden, flip and prepare on the opposite side similarly. Organize on a platter and serve them.

Almond Spinach Balls

Ingredients:

- ¼ tsp. nutmeg, ground
- 1/3 mug parmesan, grated
- Table salt and black pepper to the taste
- 1 tablespoon onion grinding grains
- 3 tbsp whipping cream
- 4 tbsp melted ghee
- 2 eggs
- 1 mug almond flour
- 16 ounces spinach
- 1/3 mug feta cheese, crumbled
- 1 tsp. garlic grinding grains

Instructions:

- In your blender, combine spinach with ghee, eggs, almond flour, feta cheese, parmesan, nutmeg, whipping cream, table salt, pepper, onion and garlic pepper and blend very well.
- Shift to a pot and keep in the freezer for 10 minutes Shape 30 spinach balls, organize on a lined baking sheet, introduce in the oven at 350 degrees F and bake for 12 minutes. Leave spinach balls to cool down and serve as a party appetizer.

Garlic Black Pepper Spinach Dip

Ingredients:

- 1 and ½ tbsp parsley, sliced off
- 2.5 ounces parmesan, grated
- 1 tablespoon lemon juice
- 6 bacon slices
- 5 ounces spinach
- ½ mug sour cream
- 8 ounces cream cheese, soft
- Table salt and black pepper to the taste
- 1 tablespoon garlic, chopped

Instructions:

- Warm up a dish over moderate heat, insert bacon, prepare until it's crispy, shift to paper towels, drain grease, crumble and leave aside in a very pot.
- Warm up the identical dish with the bacon grease over moderate heat, insert spinach, shake, prepare for two minutes and shift to a pot. In another pot, combine cream cheese with garlic, table salt, pepper, sour cream and parsley and shake well. Insert bacon and shake again. Insert lemon juice and spinach and shake everything.

- Insert parmesan and shake again. Distribute this into ramekins, introduce in the oven at 350 degrees f and bake for 25 minutes. Turn oven to broil and broil for 4 minutes more. Serve with crackers.

Mushrooms Onion Appetizer

Ingredients:

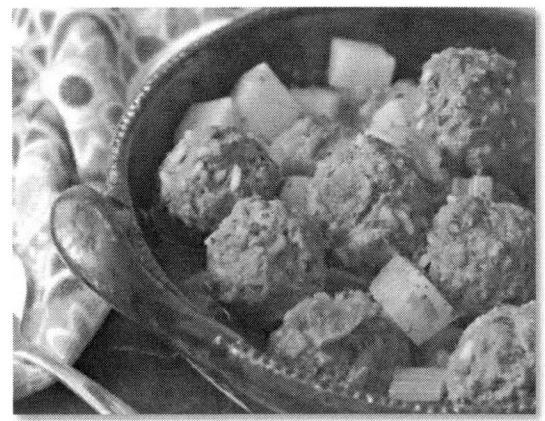

- Table salt and black pepper to the taste
- 1 tsp. curry grinding grains
- 4 ounces cream cheese, soft
- ¼ mug sour cream
- ½ mug Mexican cheese, shredded
- ¼ mug mayo
- 1 tsp. garlic grinding grains
- 1 small yellow onion, sliced off
- 24 ounces white mushroom caps
- 1 mug shrimp, prepared, peeled, deveined and sliced off

Instructions:

- In a pot, combine mayo with garlic grinding grains, onion, curry grinding grains, cream cheese, sour cream, Mexican cheese, shrimp, table salt and pepper to the taste and whisk well.
- Stuff mushrooms with this combine, put on a baking sheet and prepare in the oven at 350 degrees F for 20 minutes. Organize on a platter and serve.

Mexican Basil Meatballs

Ingredients:

- 1-pound turkey meat, ground
- ½ tsp. garlic grinding grains
- 2 tbsp sun-dried tomatoes, sliced off
- ½ mug mozzarella cheese, shredded
- 2 tbsp olive oil
- 1 egg
- Table salt and black pepper to the taste
- ¼ mug almond flour
- 2 tablespoon basil, sliced off

Instructions:

- In a pot, combine turkey with table salt, pepper, egg, almond flour, garlic grinding grains, sun-dried tomatoes, mozzarella and basil and shake well. Shape twelve meatballs, Warm up a dish with the oil over moderate immense heat, drop meatballs and prepare them for two minutes on every facet. Organize on a platter and serve.

Parmesan Chicken Wings

Ingredients:

- 2 tbsp ghee
- ½ mug parmesan cheese, grated
- A pinch of red pepper flakes, crushed
- 1 tsp. garlic grinding grains
- 6-pound chicken wings, slice in halves
- Table salt and black pepper to the taste
- ½ tsp. Italian seasoning
- 1 egg

Instructions:

- Organize chicken wings on a lined baking sheet, introduce inside the oven at 425 degrees F and bake for 17 minutes.
- Meanwhile, in your blender, combine ghee with cheese, egg, table salt, pepper, pepper flakes, garlic grinding grains and Italian seasoning and mix very well. Take chicken wings out of the oven, flip them, flip oven to broil and broil them for five minutes a heap of.
- Take chicken things out of the oven once additional, pour sauce over them, fling to coat well and broil for 1 minute additional. Serve them as a fast appetizer.

Breadcrumbs Broccoli Sticks

Ingredients:

- 1/3 mug disk breadcrumbs
- 1/3 mug Italian breadcrumbs
- 2 tbsp parsley, sliced off
- A drizzle of olive oil
- 1 egg
- 2 mugs broccoli florets
- 1/3 mug cheddar cheese, grated
- ¼ mug yellow onion, sliced off
- Table salt and black pepper to the taste

Instructions:

- Warm up a pot with water over moderate heat, insert broccoli, steam for one minute, drain, chop and put into a pot. Insert egg, cheddar cheese, disk and Italian breadcrumbs, table salt, pepper and parsley and shake everything well.
- Shape stands proud of this combine using your hands and Put them on a baking sheet which you've got greased with some olive oil. Introduce within the oven at 400 degrees F and bake for twenty minutes. Organize on a platter and serve.

Taco Table salted Mugs

Ingredients:

- Table salt and black pepper to the taste
- 2 tbsp cumin
- 2 tbsp chili grinding grains
- 1-pound beef, ground
- 2 mugs cheddar cheese, shredded
- ¼ mug water
- Pico de Gallo for serving

Instructions:

- Disseminate spoonful of parmesan on a lined preparing sheet, present in the stove at 350 degrees F and heat for seven minutes.
- Leave cheddar to chill off put for 1 moment, move them to small mug cake forms and shape them into mugs. In the interim, Warm up a dish over moderate tremendous warmth, embed hamburger, shake and plan till it tans.
- Addition the water, table salt, pepper, cumin and stew pounding grains, shake and plan for 5 minutes. Convey into cheddar mugs, top with Pico de Gallo, move all to a platter and serve.

Cucumber Mugs

Ingredients:

- Table salt and white pepper to the taste
- 6 ounces smoked salmon, flaked
- 1/3 mug cilantro, sliced off
- 2 teaspoons lime juice
- 2 cucumbers, peeled, slice into ¾ inch slices and some of the seeds
- scooped out
- ½ mug sour cream
- 1 tablespoon lime zest
- A pinch of cayenne pepper

Instructions:

- In a pot combine salmon with table salt, pepper, cayenne, sour cream, lime juice and zest and cilantro and shake well.
- Fill each cucumber mug with this salmon combine, prepare on a platter and function an appetizer.

Caviar Salad

Ingredients:

- Table salt and black pepper to the taste
- 1 yellow onion, finely sliced off

- ¾ mug mayonnaise
- 8 eggs, hard-boiled, peeled and mashed with a fork
- 4 ounces black caviar
- 4 ounces red caviar
- Some toast baguette slices for serving

Instructions:

- In a pot, combine mashed eggs with mayo, table salt, pepper and onion and shake well. Scatter eggs salad on toasted baguette slices, and immense every with caviar.

Marinated Sirloin Kebabs

Ingredients:

- 2 pounds sirloin steak, slice into moderate cubes
- 4 garlic cloves, chopped
- ¼ mug lemon juice
- ½ mug olive oil
- 1 red onion, slice into chunks
- Table salt and black pepper to the taste
- 2 tbsp Dijon mustard
- 1 red bell pepper, slice into chunks
- 1 green bell pepper, slice into chunks
- 1 orange bell pepper, slice into chunks
- 2 and ½ tbsp Worcestershire sauce
- ¼ mug tamari sauce

Instructions:

- In a pot, combine Worcestershire sauce with table salt, pepper, garlic, mustard, tamari, lemon juice and oil and whisk very well. Insert beef, bell peppers and onion chunks to this combine, fling to coat and leave aside for a few minutes.
- Organize bell pepper, meat cubes and onion chunks on skewers alternating colors, put them on your preheated grill over moderate immense heat, prepare for 5 minutes on each aspect, shift to a platter and serve as a summer appetizer.

Mint Zucchini Rolls

Ingredients:

- 2 tbsp mint, sliced off
- 1 and 1/3 mug ricotta cheese
- Table salt and black pepper to the taste
- ¼ mug basil, sliced off
- 2 tbsp olive oil
- 3 zucchinis, thinly sliced
- 24 basil leaves

- Tomato sauce for serving

Instructions:

- Brush zucchini slices with the olive oil, season with table salt and pepper on each side, put them on preheated grill over moderate heat, prepare them for two minutes, flip and prepare for 2 minutes. Put zucchini slices on a plate and leave aside for currently.
- In a pot, combine ricotta with sliced off basil, mint, table salt and pepper and shake well. Scatter this over zucchini slices, distribute whole basil leaves furthermore, roll and serve as an appetizer with some tomato sauce on the side.

Lean and Green Crackers

Ingredients:

- ½ bunch celery, sliced off
- 4 garlic cloves, chopped
- 1/3 mug olive oil
- 2 mugs flax seed, ground
- 2 mugs flax seed, soaked overnight and drained
- 4 bunches kale, sliced off
- 1 bunch basil, sliced off

Instructions:

- In your food processor combine ground flaxseed with celery, kale, basil and garlic and blend well. Insert oil and soaked flaxseed and blend once more.
- Scatter this on a tray, slice into moderate crackers, introduce in your dehydrator and dry for 24 hours at a hundred- and fifteen-degrees F, turning them halfway. Organize them on a platter and serve.

Almond Butter Bars

Ingredients:

- 1 mug almond butter
- 2 tbsp almond butter
- 4.5 ounces dark chocolate, sliced off
- 2 tbsp coconut oil
- ¾ mug coconut, unsweetened and shredded
- ¾ mug almond butter
- ¾ mug stevia

Instructions:

- In a pot, join almond flour with stevia and coconut and shake well. Warm up a dish over moderate-low warmth, embed 1 mug almond spread and hence the coconut oil and whisk well. Supplement this to almond flour and shake well. Move this to a preparing dish and press well.

- Warm up another dish with the chocolate shake ring ordinarily. Supplement the remainder of the almond margarine and whisk well again. Pour this over almond consolidate and Scatter equitably. Present inside the cooler for two hours, cut into twelve bars and fill in as a nibble.

Avocado Jalapeno Salsa

Ingredients:

- Table salt and black pepper to the taste
- 2 tbsp cumin grinding grains
- 2 tbsp lime juice
- ½ tomato, sliced off
- 1 small red onion, sliced off
- 2 avocados, pitted, peeled and sliced off
- 3 jalapeno pepper, sliced off

Instructions:

- In a pot, combine onion with avocados, peppers, table salt, black pepper, cumin, lime juice and tomato items and shake well. Shift this to a pot and serve with toasted baguette slices as an appetizer.

Almond Meal Corndogs

Ingredients:

- 1 tsp. baking grinding grains
- 1 tsp. Italian seasoning
- 2 eggs
- ½ tsp. turmeric
- 1 and ½ mugs olive oil
- 2 tbsp heavy cream
- 1 mug almond meal
- 4 sausages
- Table salt and black pepper to the taste
- A pinch of cayenne pepper

Instructions:

- In a pot, combine almond meal with Italian seasoning, baking grinding grains, turmeric, table salt, pepper and cayenne and shake well. In another pot, combine eggs with heavy cream and whisk well. Combine the two combinators and shake well.
- Dip sausages during this combine and Put them on a plate. Warm up a dish with the oil over moderate immense heat, insert sausages, prepare for two minutes on each side and shift to paper towels. Drain grease, organize on a platter and serve.

Chili Lime Chips

Ingredients:

- 1 and ½ teaspoons lime zest
- 1 tsp. lime juice
- 1 egg
- 1 mug almond flour
- Table salt and black pepper to the taste

Instructions:

- In a pot, combine almond flour with lime zest, lime juice and table salt and shake. Insert egg and whisk well once more.
- Distribute this into four elements, roll each into a ball and then Scatter well using a rolling pin. Slice each into vi triangles, put them all on a lined baking sheet, introduce within the oven at 350 degrees F and bake for twenty minutes.

Roasted Onion Garlic Dip

Ingredients:

- 1 large, sweet onion, peeled and cut into eighths
- 8 garlic cloves
- 2 teaspoons olive oil
- ½ cup light sour cream
- 1 tablespoon fresh lemon juice
- 1 tablespoon chopped fresh parsley
- 1 teaspoon chopped fresh thyme
- Freshly ground black pepper

Instructions:

- Preheat the oven to 425°F.
- In a small bowl, toss the onion and garlic with the olive oil.
- Transfer the onion and garlic to a piece of aluminum foil and wrap the
- vegetables loosely in a packet.
- Place the foil packet on a small baking sheet and place the sheet in the
- oven.
- Roast the vegetables for 50 minutes to 1 hour, or until they are very fragrant
- and golden.
- Remove the packet from the oven and allow it to cool for 15 minutes.
- In a medium bowl, stir together the sour cream, lemon juice, parsley,
- thyme, and black pepper.
- Open the foil packet carefully and transfer the vegetables to a cutting board.
- Chop the vegetables and add them to the sour cream mixture. Stir to
- combine.
- Cover the dip and chill in the refrigerator for 1 hour before serving.

Baba Ghanoush

Ingredients:

- 1 medium eggplant, halved and scored with a crosshatch pattern on the cut sides
- 1 tablespoon olive oil, plus extra for brushing
- 1 large, sweet onion, peeled and diced
- 2 garlic cloves, halved
- 1 teaspoon ground cumin
- 1 teaspoon ground coriander
- 1 tablespoon lemon juice
- Freshly ground black pepper

Instructions:

- Preheat the oven to 400°F.
- Line 2 baking sheets with parchment paper.
- Brush the eggplant halves with olive oil and place them, cut side down, on 1 baking sheet.
- In a small bowl, mix together the onion, garlic, 1 tablespoon olive oil, cumin, and coriander.
- Spread the seasoned onions on the other baking sheet.
- Place both baking sheets in the oven and roast the onions for about 20 minutes and the eggplant for 30 minutes, or until softened and browned.
- Remove the vegetables from the oven and scrape the eggplant flesh into a bowl.
- Transfer the onions and garlic to a cutting board and chop coarsely; add to
- the eggplant.
- Stir in the lemon juice and pepper.
- Serve warm or chilled.

Spicy Kale Chips

Ingredients:

- 2 cups kale
- 2 teaspoons olive oil
- ¼ teaspoon chili powder
- Pinch cayenne pepper

Instructions:

- Preheat the oven to 300°F.
- Line 2 baking sheets with parchment paper; set aside.
- Remove the stems from the kale and tear the leaves into 2-inch pieces.
- Wash the kale and dry it completely.
- Transfer the kale to a large bowl and drizzle with olive oil.
- Use your hands to toss the kale with the oil, taking care to coat each leaf evenly.
- Season the kale with chili powder and cayenne pepper and toss to combine thoroughly.
- Spread the seasoned kale in a single layer on each baking sheet. Do not overlap the leaves.
- Bake the kale, rotating the pans once, for 20 to 25 minutes or until it is crisp and dry.
- Remove the trays from the oven and allow the chips to cool on the trays for 5 minutes.
- Serve immediately.

Cinnamon Tortilla Chips

Ingredients:

- 2 teaspoons granulated sugar
- ½ teaspoon ground cinnamon
- Pinch ground nutmeg
- 3 (6-inch) flour tortillas
- Cooking spray, for coating the tortillas

Instructions:

- Preheat the oven to 350°F.
- Line a baking sheet with parchment paper.
- In a small bowl, stir together the sugar, cinnamon, and nutmeg.
- Lay the tortillas on a clean work surface and spray both sides of each lightly with cooking spray.
- Sprinkle the cinnamon sugar evenly over both sides of each tortilla.
- Cut the tortillas into 16 wedges each and place them on the baking sheet.
- Bake the tortilla wedges, turning once, for about 10 minutes or until crisp.
- Cool the chips and store in a sealed container at room temperature for up to 1 week.

Sweet and Spicy Kettle Corn

Ingredients:

- 3 tablespoons olive oil
- 1 cup popcorn kernels
- ½ cup brown sugar
- Pinch cayenne pepper

Instructions:

- Place a large pot with lid over medium heat and add the olive oil with a few popcorn kernels.
- Shake the pot lightly until the popcorn kernels pop. Add the rest of the kernels and sugar to the pot.
- Pop the kernels with the lid on the pot, shaking constantly, until they are all popped.
- Remove the pot from the heat and transfer the popcorn to a large bowl.
- Toss the popcorn with the cayenne pepper and serve.

Blueberries and Cream Ice Pops

Ingredients:

- 3 cups fresh blueberries
- 1 teaspoon freshly squeezed lemon juice
- ¼ cup unsweetened rice milk
- ¼ cup light sour cream
- ¼ cup granulated sugar
- ½ teaspoon pure vanilla extract
- ¼ teaspoon ground cinnamon

Instructions:

- Put the blueberries, lemon juice, rice milk, sour cream, sugar, vanilla, and
- cinnamon in a blender and purée until smooth.
- Spoon the mixture into ice-pop molds and freeze for 3 to 4 hours or until very firm.

Meringue Cookies
Ingredients:

- 4 egg whites, at room temperature
- 1 cup granulated sugar
- 1 teaspoon pure vanilla extract
- 1 teaspoon almond extract
- Preheat the oven to 300°F.
- Line 2 baking sheets with parchment; set aside.

Instructions:

- In a large stainless-steel bowl, beat the egg whites until stiff peaks form.
- Add the granulated sugar 1 tablespoon at a time, beating well to incorporate after each addition, until all the sugar is used, and the meringue is thick and glossy.
- Beat in the vanilla extract and almond extract.
- Using a tablespoon, drop the meringue batter onto the baking sheets, spacing the cookies evenly.
- Bake the cookies for about 30 minutes or until they are crisp.
- Remove the cookies from the oven and let them cool on wire racks.
- Store the cookies in an airtight container at room temperature for up to 1 week.

- Serve warm.

Roasted Red Pepper and Chicken Crostini
Ingredients:

- 2 tablespoons olive oil
- ½ teaspoon minced garlic
- 4 slices French bread
- 1 roasted red bell pepper, chopped
- 4 ounces cooked chicken breast, shredded
- ½ cup chopped fresh basil

Instructions:

- Preheat the oven to 400°F.
- Line a baking sheet with aluminum foil.
- In a small bowl, mix together the olive oil and garlic.
- Brush both sides of each piece of bread with the olive oil mixture.
- Place the bread on the baking sheet and toast in the oven, turning once, for
- about 5 minutes or until both sides are golden and crisp.
- In a medium bowl, stir together the red pepper, chicken, and basil.
- Top each toasted bread slice with the red pepper mixture and serve.

Cucumber Wrapped Vegetable Rolls

Ingredients:

- ½ cup finely shredded red cabbage
- ½ cup grated carrot
- ¼ cup julienned red bell pepper
- ¼ cup julienned scallion, both green and white parts
- ¼ cup chopped cilantro
- 1 tablespoon olive oil
- ¼ teaspoon ground cumin
- ¼ teaspoon freshly ground black pepper
- 1 English cucumber, sliced into 8 very thin strips with a vegetable peeler

Instructions:

- In a medium bowl, toss together the cabbage, carrot, red pepper, scallion, cilantro, olive oil, cumin, and black pepper until well mixed.
- Evenly divide the vegetable filling among the cucumber strips, placing the filling close to one end of the strip.
- Roll up the cucumber strips around the filling and secure with a wooden pick.
- Repeat with each cucumber strip.

Antojitos

Ingredients:

- 6 ounces plain cream cheese, at room temperature
- ½ jalapeño pepper, finely chopped
- ½ scallion, green part only, chopped
- ¼ cup finely chopped red bell pepper
- ½ teaspoon ground cumin
- ½ teaspoon ground coriander
- ½ teaspoon chili powder
- 3 (8-inch) flour tortillas

Instructions:

- In a medium bowl, mix together the cream cheese, jalapeño pepper, scallion, red bell pepper, cumin, coriander, and chili powder until well blended.
- Divide the cream cheese mixture evenly among the 3 tortillas, spreading the cheese in a thin layer and leaving a ¼-inch edge all the way around.
- Roll the tortillas like a jelly roll and wrap each tightly in plastic wrap.
- Refrigerate the rolls for about 1 hour or until they are set.
- Cut the tortilla rolls into 1-inch pieces and arrange them on a plate to serve.

Chicken Vegetable Kebabs

Ingredients:

- 2 tablespoons olive oil
- 2 tablespoons freshly squeezed lemon juice
- ½ teaspoon minced garlic
- ½ teaspoon chopped fresh thyme

- 4 ounces boneless, skinless chicken breast, cut into 8 pieces
- 1 small summer squash, cut into 8 pieces
- ½ medium onion, cut into 8 pieces

Instructions:

- In a medium bowl, stir together the olive oil, lemon juice, garlic, and thyme.
- Add the chicken to the bowl and stir to coat.
- Cover the bowl with plastic wrap and place the chicken in the refrigerator to marinate for 1 hour.
- Thread the squash, onion, and chicken pieces onto 4 large skewers, evenly dividing the vegetables and meat among the skewers.
- Heat a barbecue to medium and grill the skewers, turning at least 2 times, for 10 to 12 minutes or until the chicken is cooked through.

Five Spice Chicken Lettuce Wraps

Ingredients:

- 6 ounces cooked chicken breast, minced
- 1 scallion, both green and white parts, chopped
- ½ red apple, cored and chopped
- ½ cup bean sprouts
- ¼ English cucumber, finely chopped
- Juice of 1 lime
- Zest of 1 lime
- 2 tablespoons chopped fresh cilantro
- ½ teaspoon Chinese five-spice powder
- 8 Boston lettuce leaves

Instructions:

- In a large bowl, mix together the chicken, scallions, apple, bean sprouts, cucumber, lime juice, lime zest, cilantro, and five-spice powder.
- Spoon the chicken mixture evenly among the 8 lettuce leaves.
- Wrap the lettuce around the chicken mixture and serve.

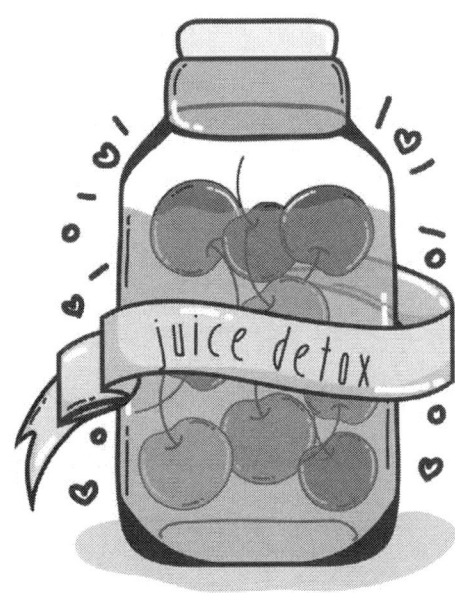

Chapter 6: Smoothies and Drinks

Berry Smoothie
Ingredients:

- ¼ cup cranberry juice cocktail
- 2/3 cup silken tofu, firm
- ½ cup raspberries, frozen, unsweetened
- ½ cup blueberries, frozen, unsweetened
- 1 teaspoon vanilla extract

Instructions:

- Pour juice into a blender. Add rest of ingredients. Blend until very smooth. Serve immediately and enjoy!

Banana Apple Smoothie
Ingredients:

- ½ banana, peeled and cut into chunks
- ½ cup plain yogurt
- ½ cup applesauce, unsweetened
- ¼ cup almond or rice milk
- 1 tablespoon honey
- 2 tablespoons oat or wheat bran

Instructions:

- Place banana, yogurt, applesauce, milk and honey in blender. Blend until smooth. Add oat bran and blend until thickened.

Kidney Cleanser Juice

Ingredients:

- 1 cup organic cranberries
- 4 cups of filtered water, divided
- 4 dates or 2 Tbsp. date paste or 2 Tbsp. maple syrup
- 2 red organic apples, sliced
- Juice of 2 organic lemons
- 1 Tsp. Cardamom (optional)
- 1 sprig fresh organic mint or peppermint (optional)

Instructions:

- In a medium size pot combine the cranberries and 3 cups of water and bring to a boil. Turn the heat off and let cool. In a food processor blend the dates or date paste with lemon juice and remaining one cup of water. Transfer to a large glass container or jar and add sliced apples, and all the cranberries and water. Stir and add cardamom and mint leaves if desired.

Blueberry Blast Smoothie

Ingredients:

- 1 cup frozen blueberries
- 8 packets of Splenda®
- 6 tablespoons of protein powder
- 8 ice cubes
- 14 ounces of apple juice (no added sugar)

Instructions:

- Place all ingredients in a blender and blend until smooth.

Easy Pineapple Protein Smoothie

Ingredients:

- 3/4 cup pineapple sherbet or sorbet
- 1 scoop vanilla whey protein powder
- 1/2 cup water
- 2 ice cubes, optional

Instructions:

- In a blender, add pineapple sherbet, whey protein powder and water (ice cubes optional).
- Immediately blend for 30 to 45 seconds.

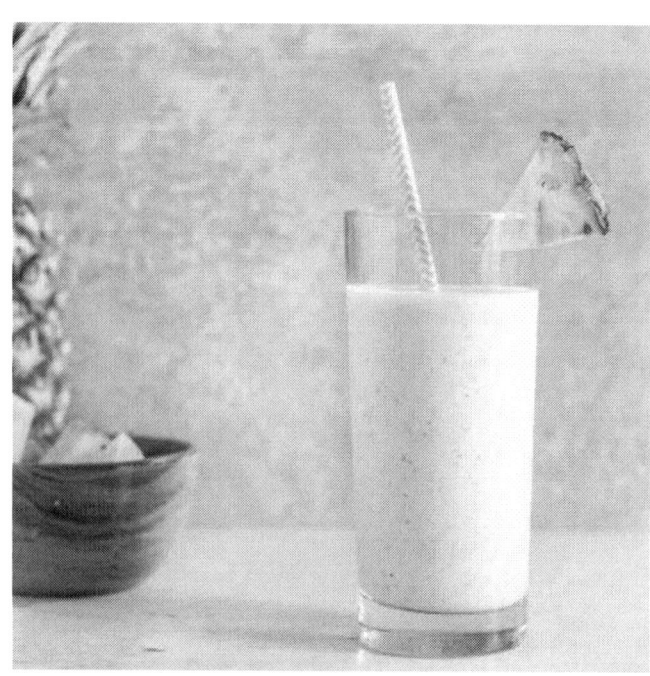

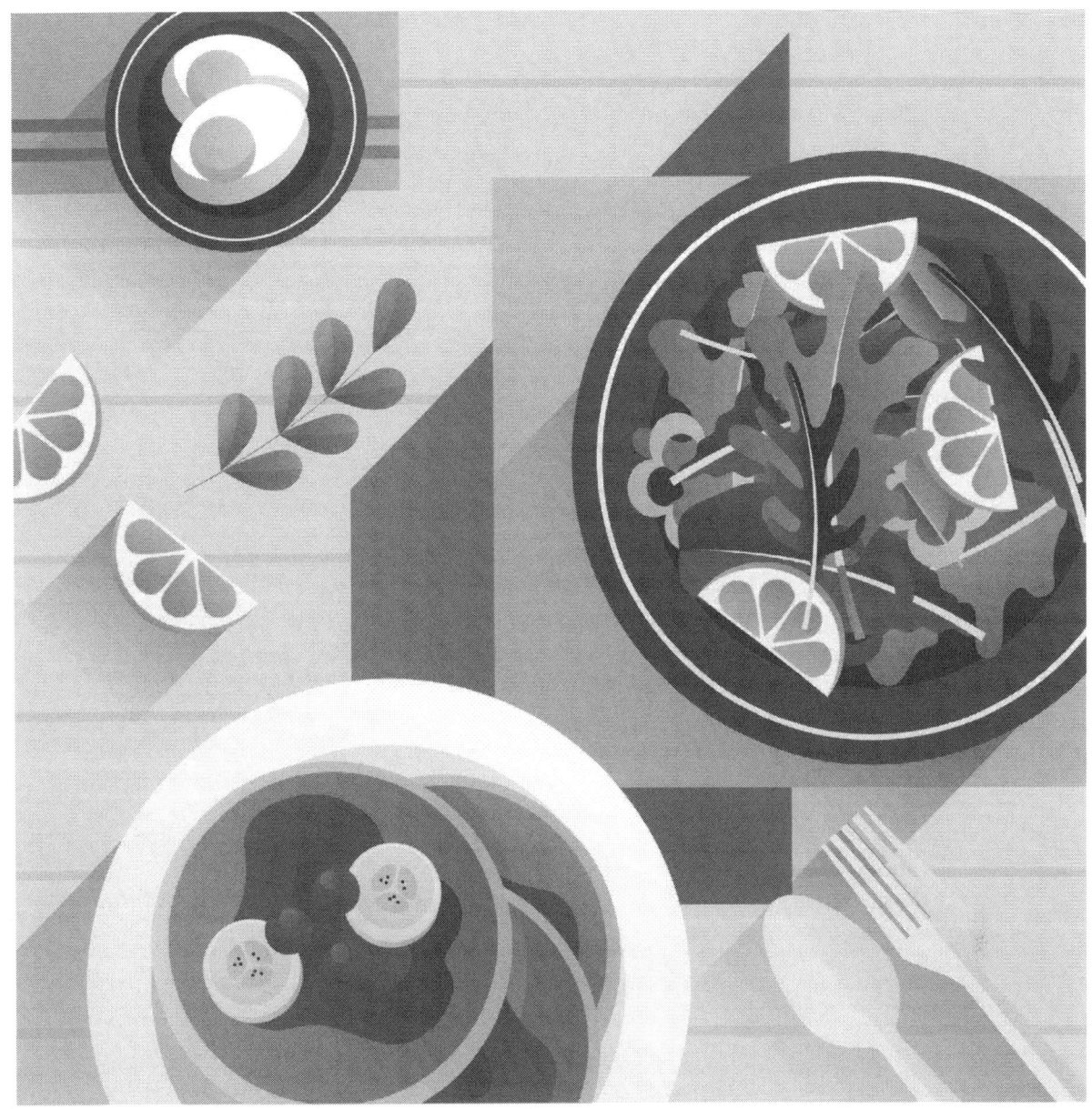

Chapter 6: Food Journal

A food journal is useful for organizing your diet and keeping track of your progress.

It is also important to combine a diet with workout that helps the body and mind. A Yoga session of a few minutes a day can also be useful to start.

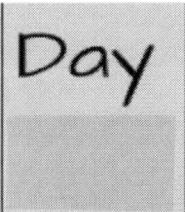 **Day**   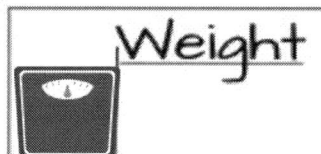 **Weight**   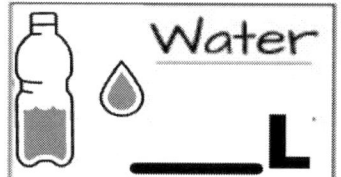 **Water** ___ L   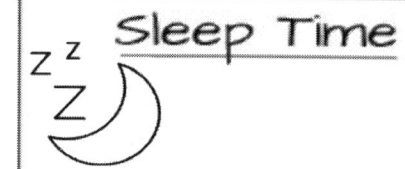 **Sleep Time**

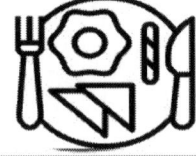 **Breakfast**

_____
_____
_____
_____

 **Lunch**

_____
_____
_____
_____

 **Dinner**

_____
_____
_____
_____

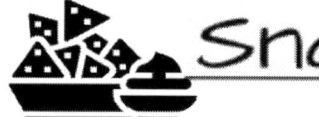 **Snacks**

_____
_____
_____
_____

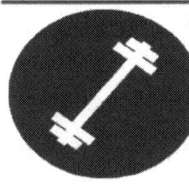 **Workout**

_____
_____
_____

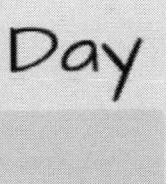 **Day** 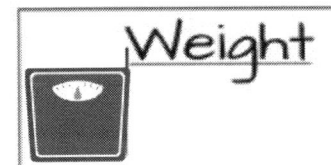 **Weight** 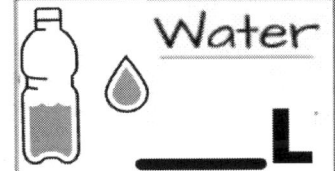 **Water** ___ **L** 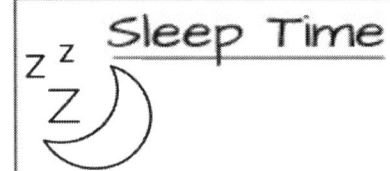 **Sleep Time**

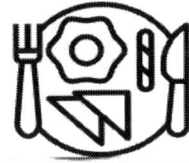 **Breakfast** _____

 **Lunch** _____

 **Dinner** _____

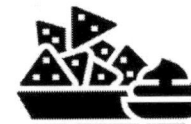 **Snacks** _____

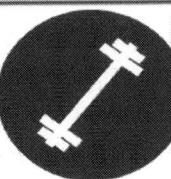 **Workout** _____

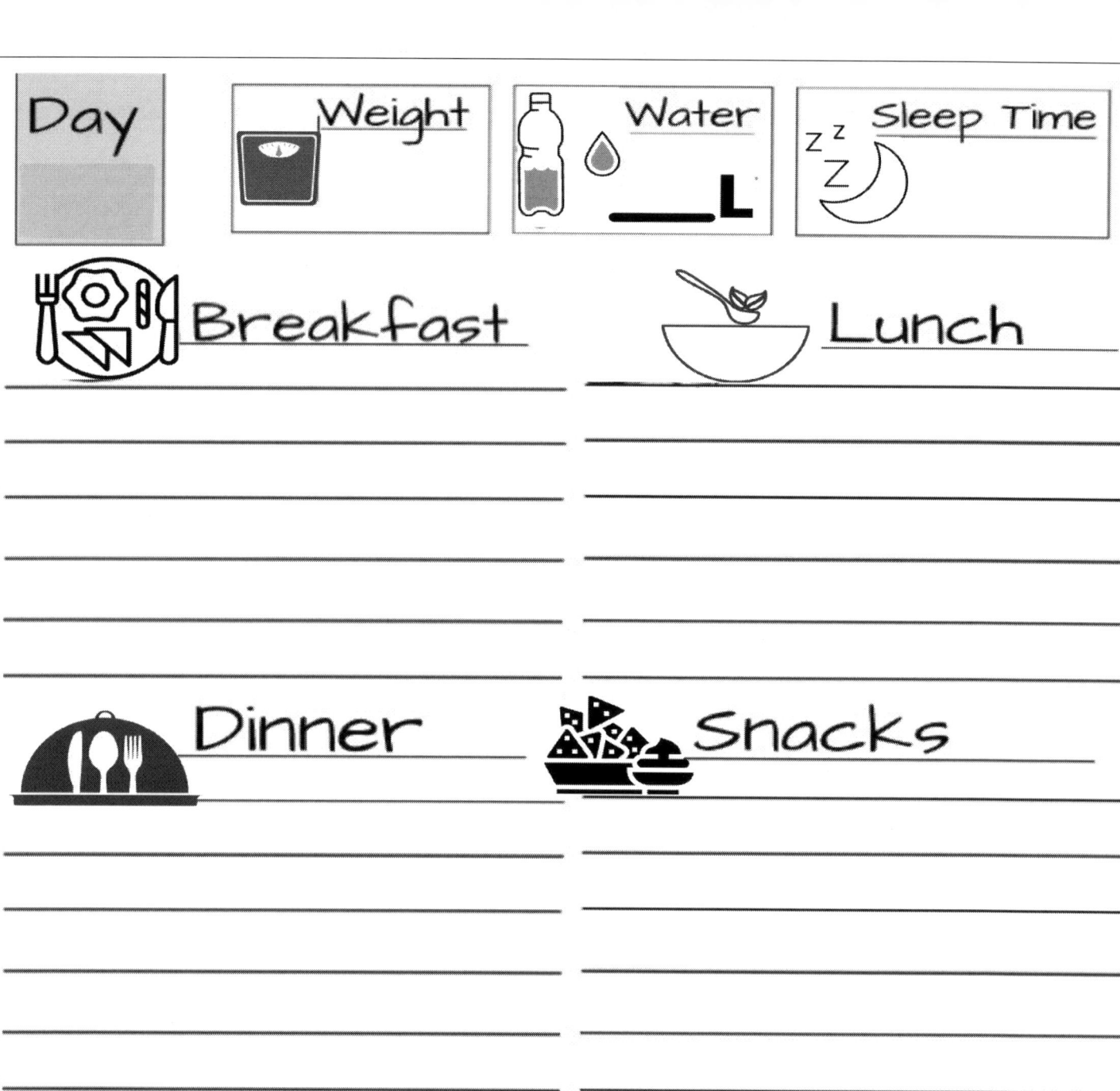

Day

Weight

Water ___L

Sleep Time

Breakfast

Lunch

Dinner

Snacks

Workout

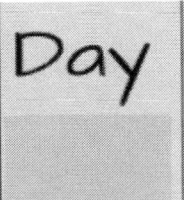 **Day** 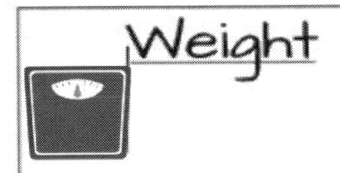 **Weight** 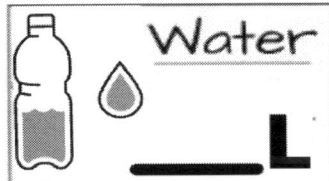 **Water** ____ L 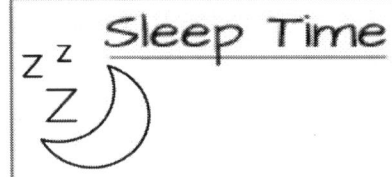 **Sleep Time**

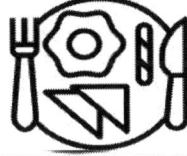 **Breakfast** ____

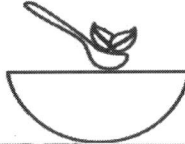 **Lunch** ____

 **Dinner** ____

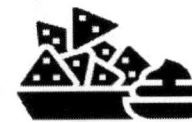 **Snacks** ____

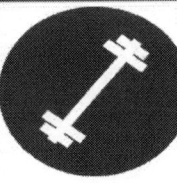 **Workout** ____

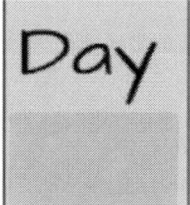 **Day**

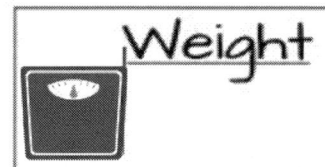 **Weight**

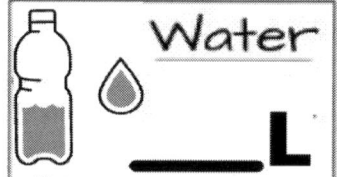 **Water** ___ **L**

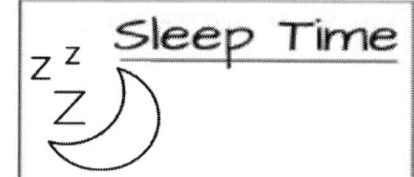 **Sleep Time**

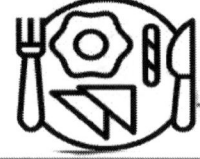 **Breakfast** ___

_____
_____
_____
_____
_____

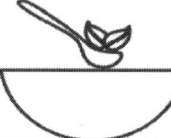 **Lunch** ___

_____
_____
_____
_____
_____

 **Dinner** ___

_____
_____
_____
_____

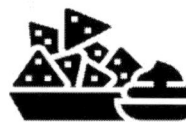 **Snacks** ___

_____
_____
_____
_____

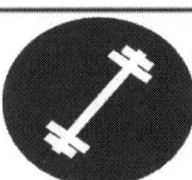 **Workout** ___

_____
_____
_____

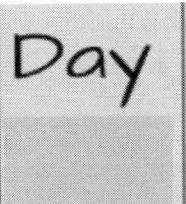 **Day**

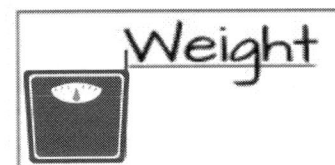 **Weight**

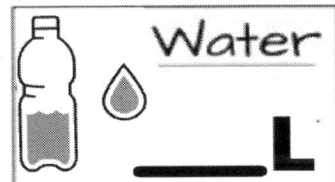 **Water** ___ **L**

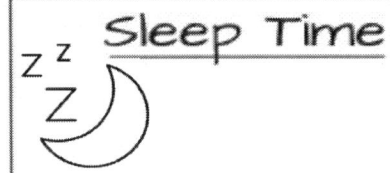 **Sleep Time**

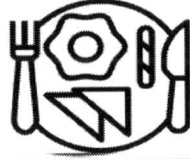 **Breakfast**

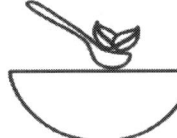 **Lunch**

 **Dinner**

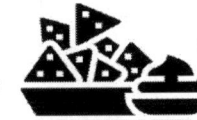 **Snacks**

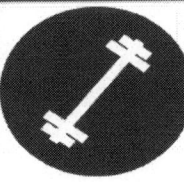 **Workout**

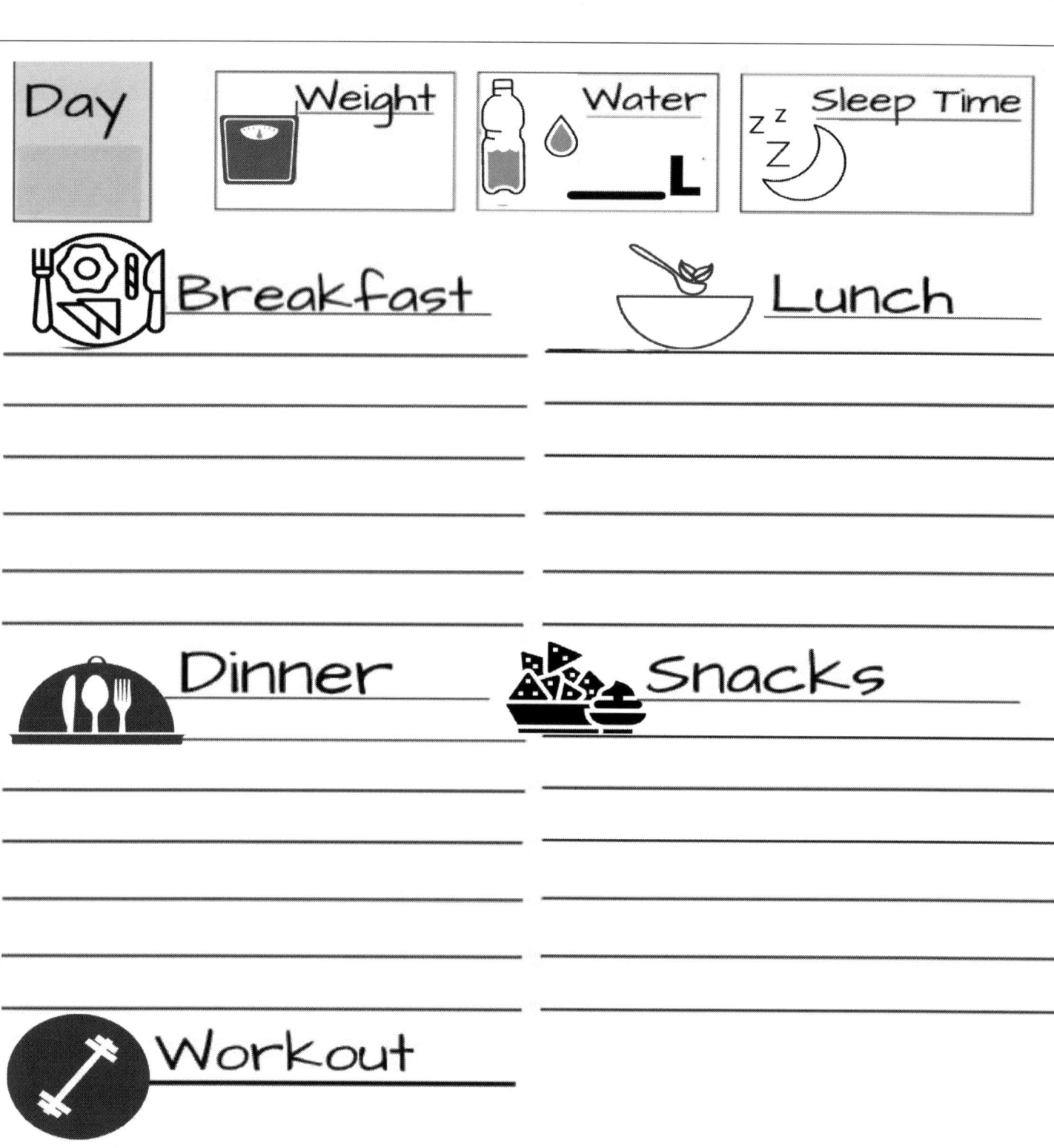

Day

Weight

Water ___L

Sleep Time

Breakfast

Lunch

Dinner

Snacks

Workout

 **Day** 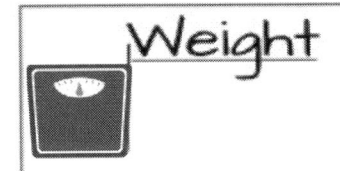 **Weight** 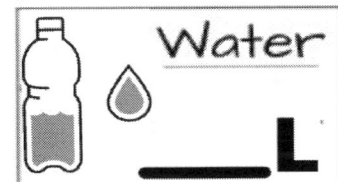 **Water** ___L 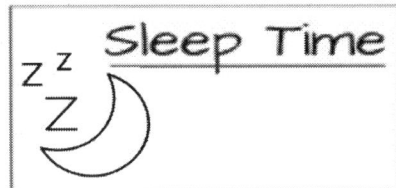 **Sleep Time**

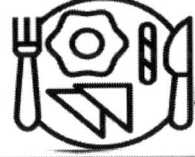 **Breakfast**

_____

_____

_____

_____

_____

 **Lunch**

_____

_____

_____

_____

_____

_____

 **Dinner**

_____

_____

_____

_____

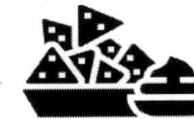 **Snacks**

_____

_____

_____

_____

_____

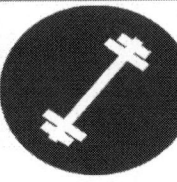 **Workout**

_____

_____

_____

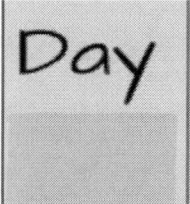 **Day**
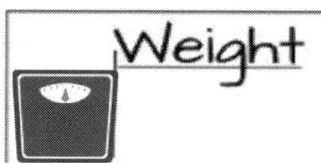 **Weight**
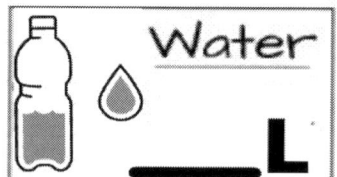 **Water** ___L
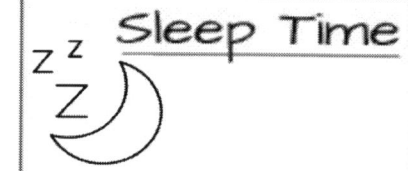 **Sleep Time**

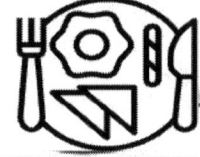 **Breakfast** _____

_____
_____
_____
_____

 **Lunch** _____

_____
_____
_____
_____

 **Dinner** _____

_____
_____
_____
_____

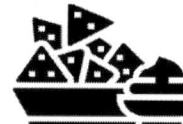 **Snacks** _____

_____
_____
_____
_____

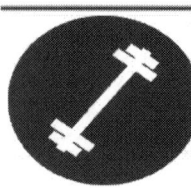 **Workout** _____

_____
_____
_____

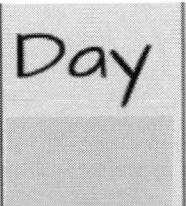 **Day** 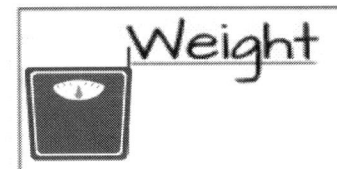 **Weight** 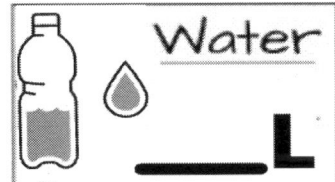 **Water** ____ **L** 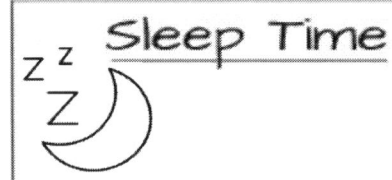 **Sleep Time**

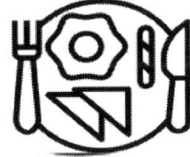 Breakfast

 Lunch

 Dinner

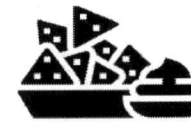 Snacks

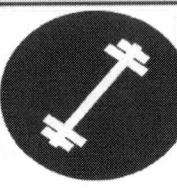 Workout

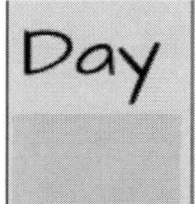 **Day**

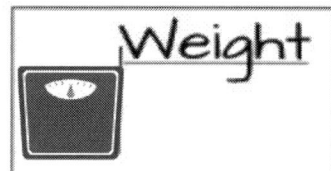 **Weight**

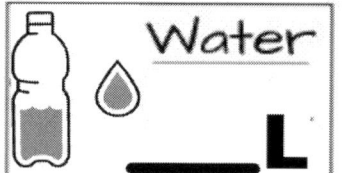 **Water** ____L

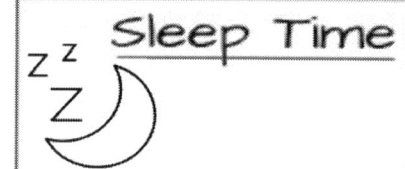 **Sleep Time**

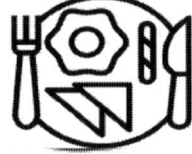 **Breakfast**

_____

_____

_____

_____

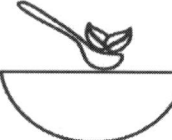 **Lunch**

_____

_____

_____

_____

 **Dinner**

_____

_____

_____

_____

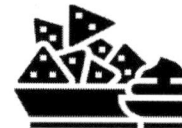 **Snacks**

_____

_____

_____

_____

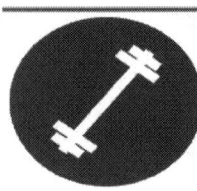 **Workout**

_____

_____

_____

 **Day**

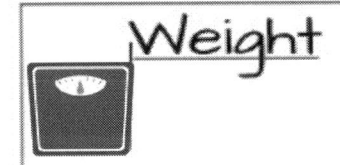 **Weight**

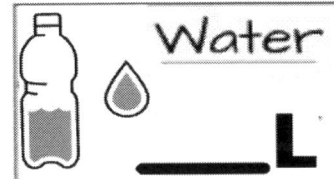 **Water** ___ **L**

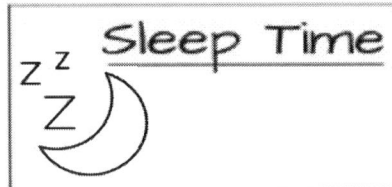 **Sleep Time**

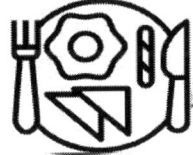 **Breakfast** _____

_____
_____
_____
_____
_____
_____

 **Lunch** _____

_____
_____
_____
_____
_____
_____

 **Dinner** _____

_____
_____
_____
_____

 **Snacks** _____

_____
_____
_____
_____

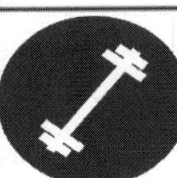 **Workout** _____

_____
_____
_____

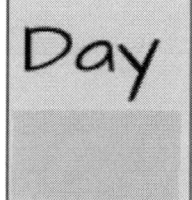 Day 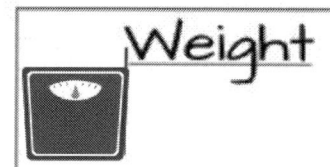 Weight 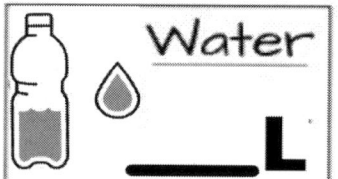 Water ___L 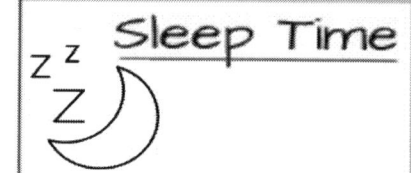 Sleep Time

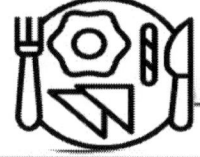 Breakfast
_____
_____
_____
_____
_____

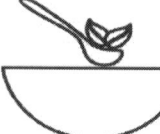 Lunch
_____
_____
_____
_____
_____

 Dinner
_____
_____
_____
_____

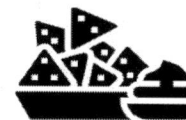 Snacks
_____
_____
_____
_____

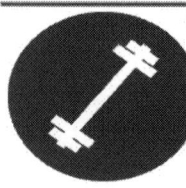 Workout
_____
_____
_____

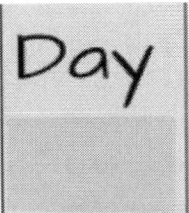 **Day**

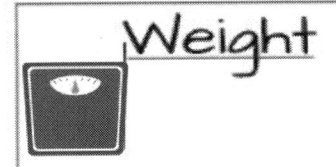 **Weight**

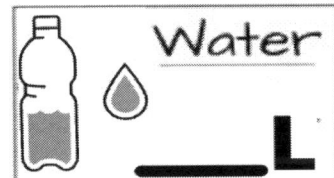 **Water** ____L

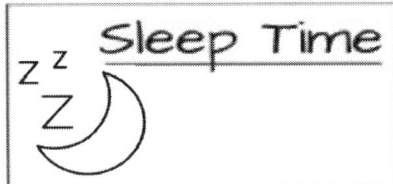 **Sleep Time**

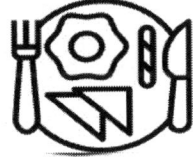 **Breakfast**

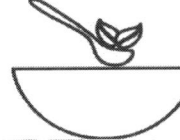 **Lunch**

 **Dinner**

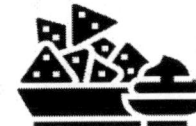 **Snacks**

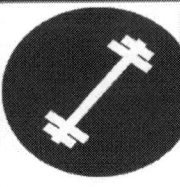 **Workout**

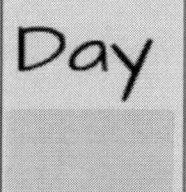 **Day**

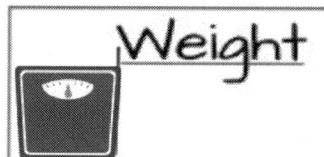 **Weight**

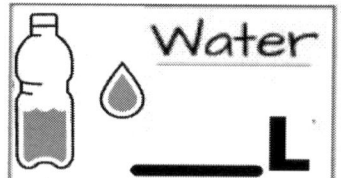 **Water** ____L

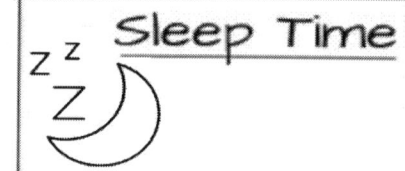 **Sleep Time**

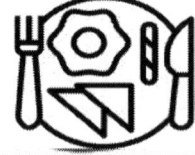 **Breakfast**

_____
_____
_____
_____
_____

 **Lunch**

_____
_____
_____
_____
_____

 **Dinner**

_____
_____
_____
_____

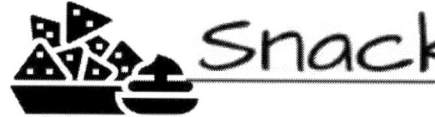 **Snacks**

_____
_____
_____
_____

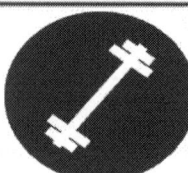 **Workout**

_____
_____
_____

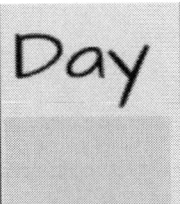 **Day** 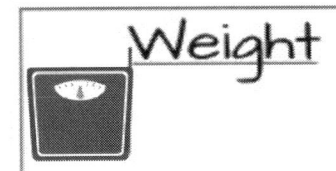 **Weight** 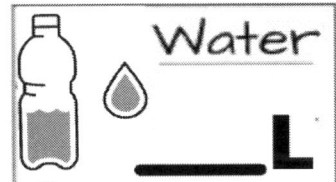 **Water** ___ **L** 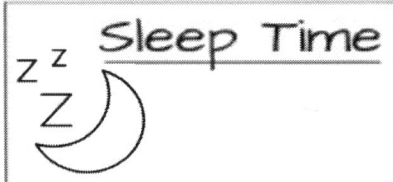 **Sleep Time**

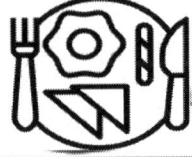 **Breakfast**

_____

_____

_____

_____

_____

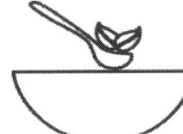 **Lunch**

_____

_____

_____

_____

_____

 **Dinner**

_____

_____

_____

_____

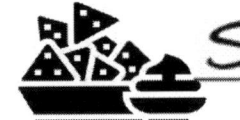 **Snacks**

_____

_____

_____

_____

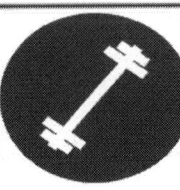 **Workout**

_____

_____

_____

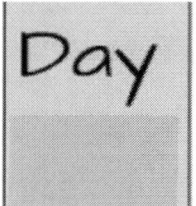 **Day**
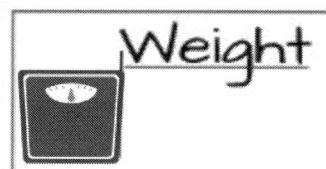 **Weight**
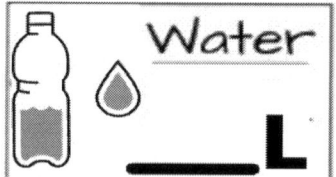 **Water** ___ **L**
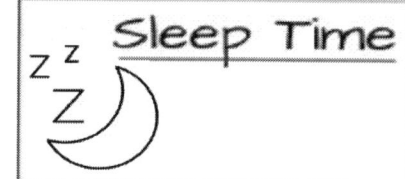 **Sleep Time**

 Breakfast

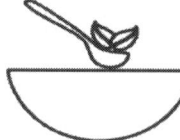 Lunch

 Dinner

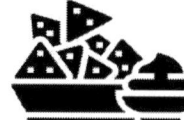 Snacks

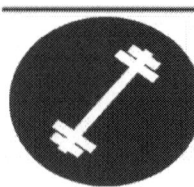 Workout

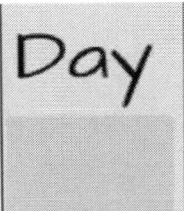 **Day**

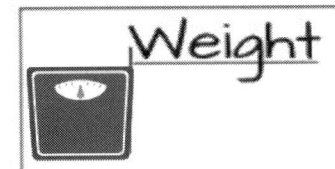 **Weight**

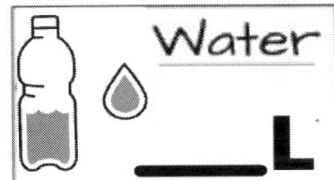 **Water** _____L

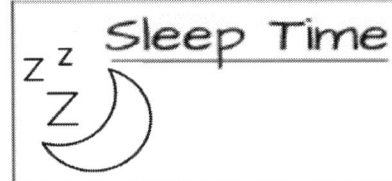 **Sleep Time**

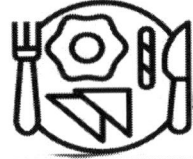 **Breakfast** _____

_____

_____

_____

_____

 **Lunch** _____

_____

_____

_____

_____

 **Dinner** _____

_____

_____

_____

_____

 **Snacks** _____

_____

_____

_____

_____

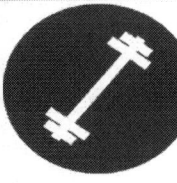 **Workout** _____

_____

_____

_____

| Day | Weight | Water ___L | Sleep Time |

Breakfast

_____
_____
_____
_____
_____

Lunch

_____
_____
_____
_____
_____

Dinner

_____
_____
_____
_____

Snacks

_____
_____
_____
_____

Workout

_____
_____
_____

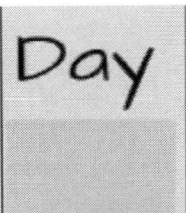 **Day** 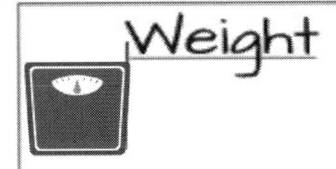 **Weight** 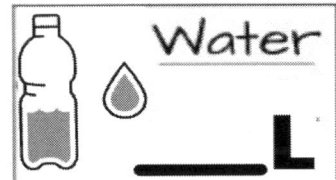 **Water** ___ **L** 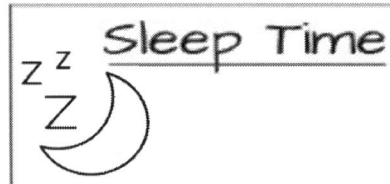 **Sleep Time**

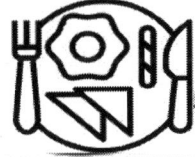 **Breakfast**

 **Lunch**

 **Dinner**

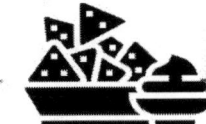 **Snacks**

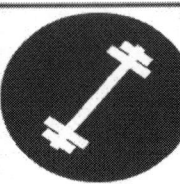 **Workout**

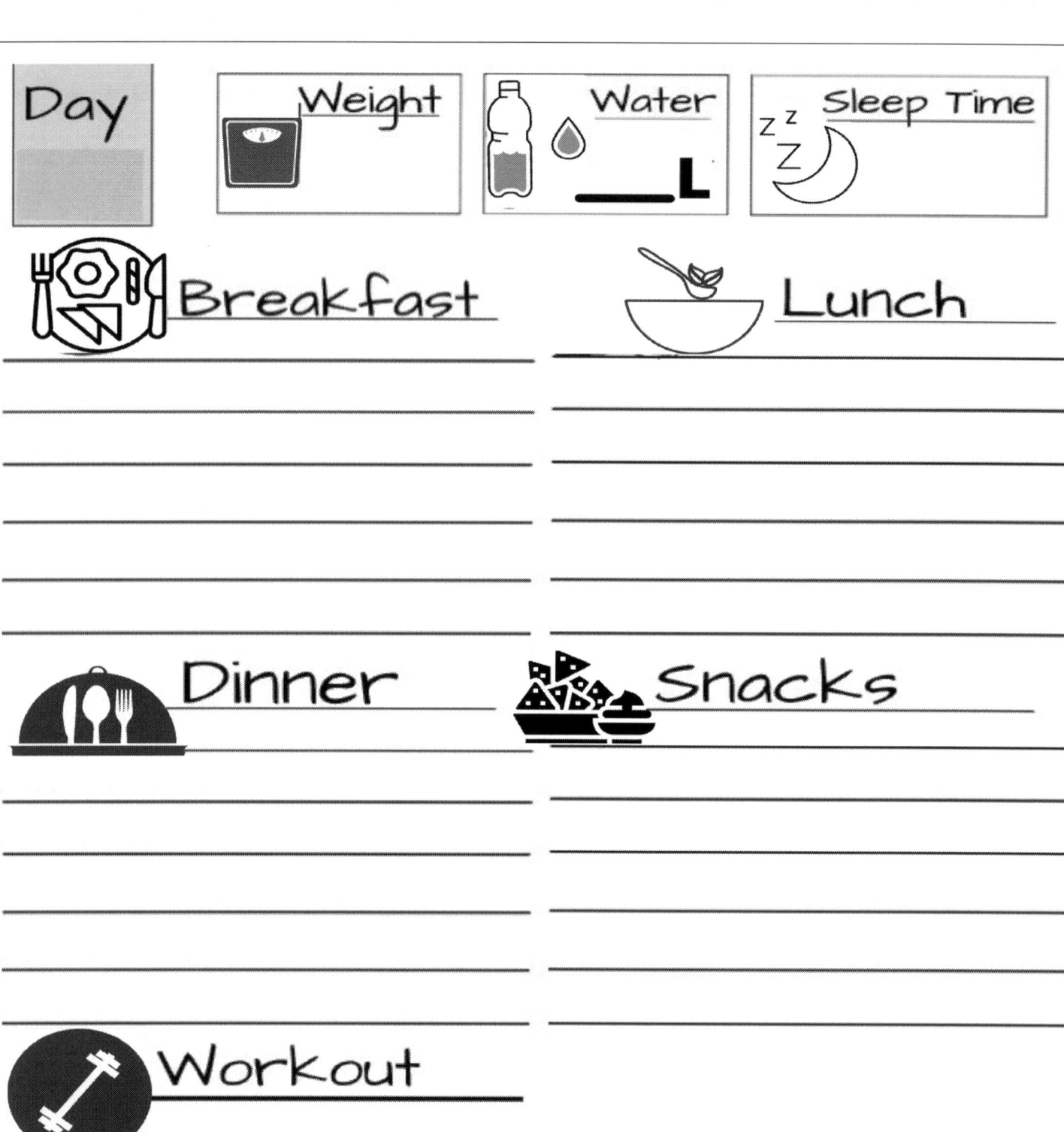

Day

Weight

Water ____ L

Sleep Time

Breakfast

Lunch

Dinner

Snacks

Workout

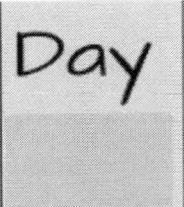 Day

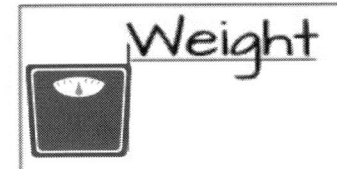 Weight

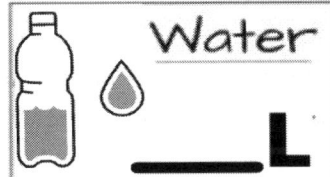 Water ___ L

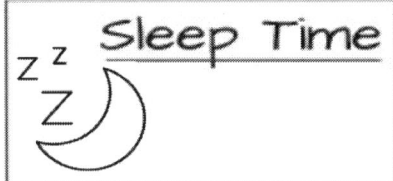 Sleep Time

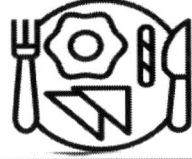 Breakfast

 Lunch

 Dinner

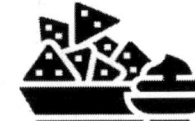 Snacks

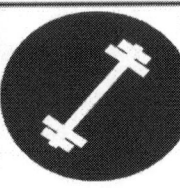 Workout

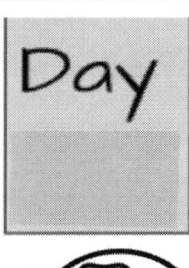 **Day**

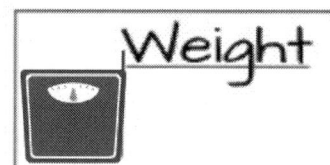 **Weight**

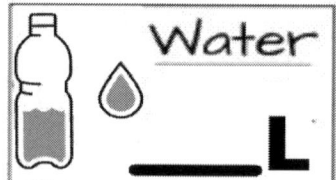 **Water** ___L

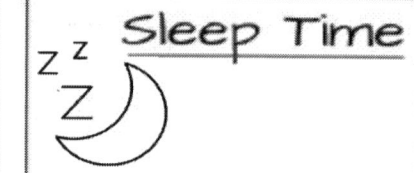 **Sleep Time**

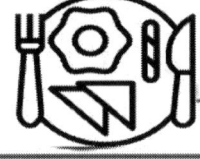 **Breakfast**

_____
_____
_____
_____
_____

 **Lunch**

_____
_____
_____
_____
_____

 **Dinner**

_____
_____
_____
_____

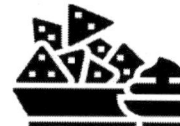 **Snacks**

_____
_____
_____
_____

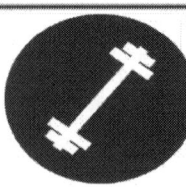 **Workout**

_____
_____
_____

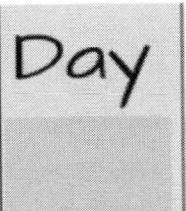 Day 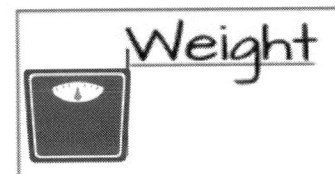 Weight 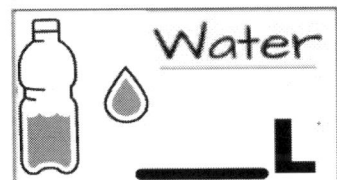 Water ___L 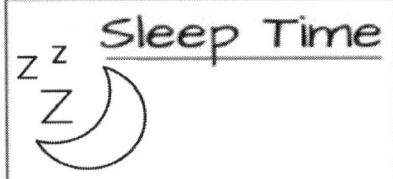 Sleep Time

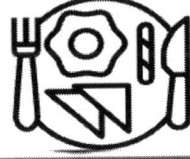 Breakfast

 Lunch

 Dinner

 Snacks

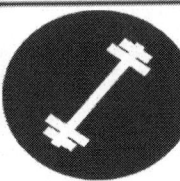 Workout

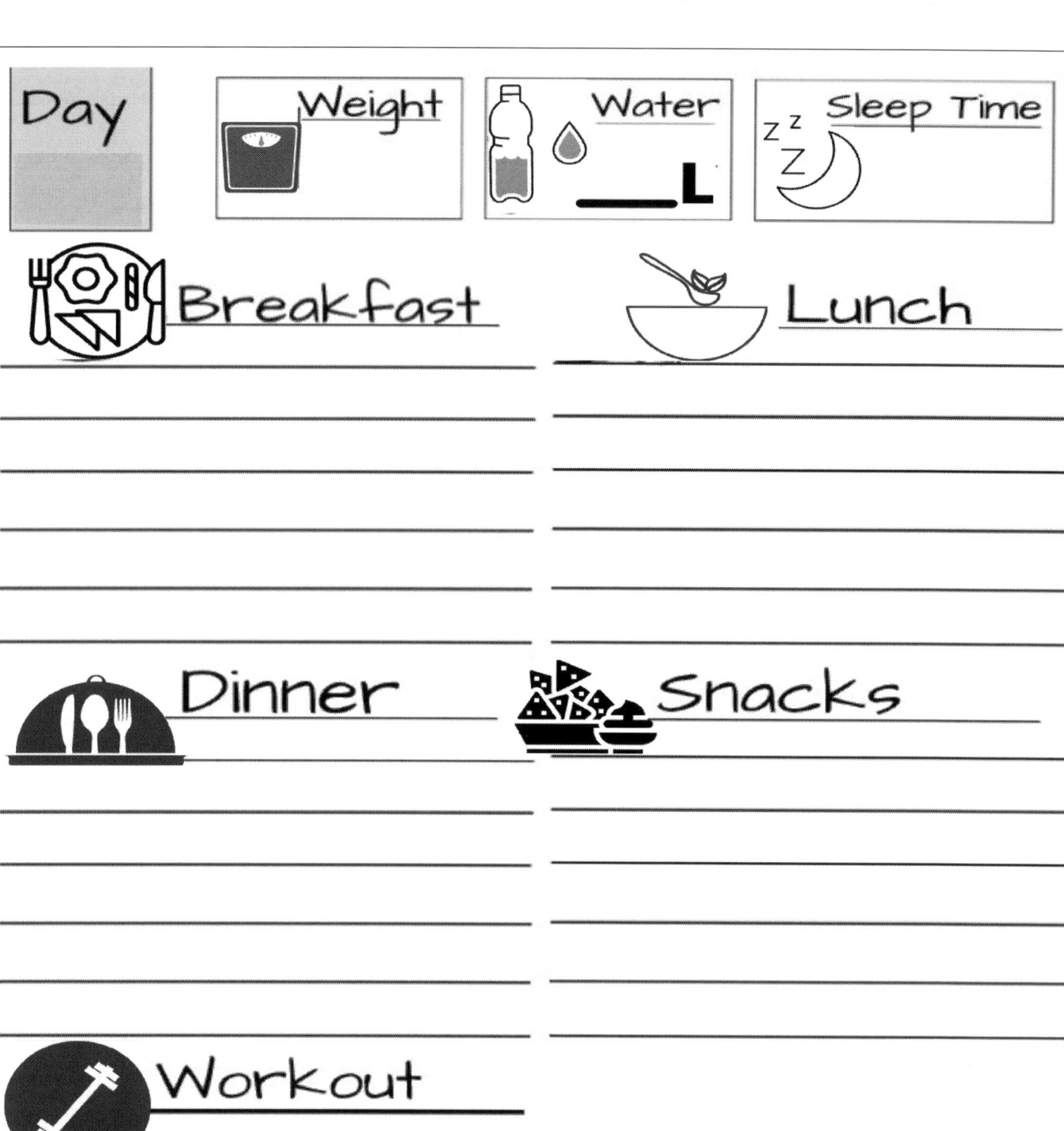

Day

Weight

Water ___ L

Sleep Time

Breakfast

Lunch

Dinner

Snacks

Workout

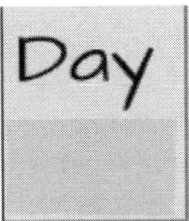 **Day** 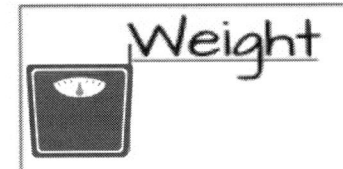 **Weight** 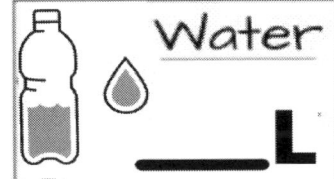 **Water** ___ **L** 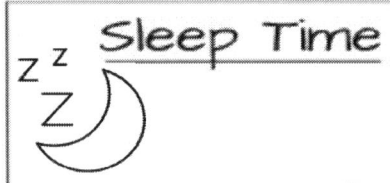 **Sleep Time**

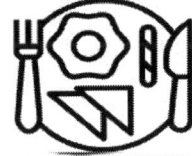 **Breakfast**

 **Lunch**

 **Dinner**

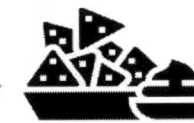 **Snacks**

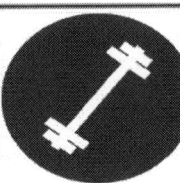 **Workout**

223

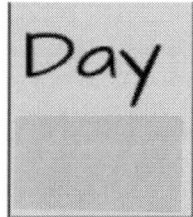 **Day**

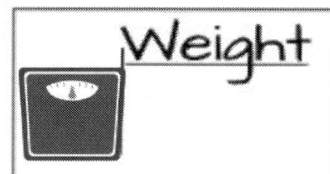 **Weight**

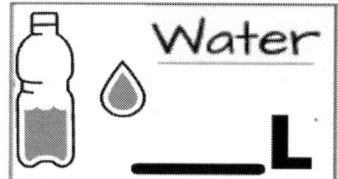 **Water** ___L

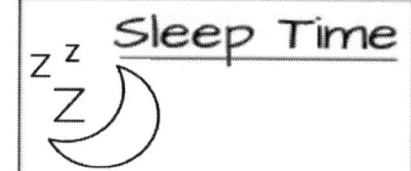 **Sleep Time**

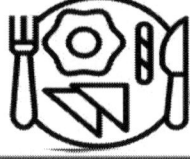 Breakfast

_____
_____
_____
_____
_____

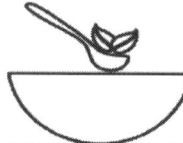 Lunch

_____
_____
_____
_____
_____

 Dinner

_____
_____
_____
_____

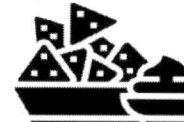 Snacks

_____
_____
_____
_____

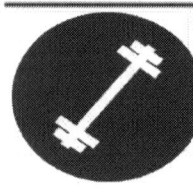 Workout

_____
_____
_____

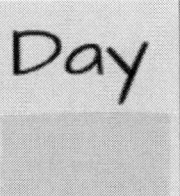 **Day**

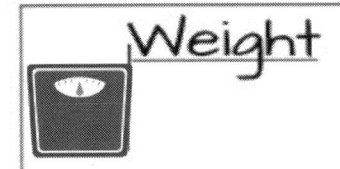 **Weight**

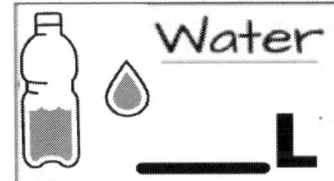 **Water** ____ **L**

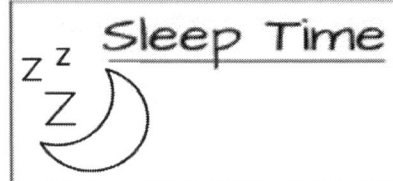 **Sleep Time**

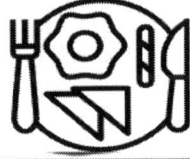 **Breakfast**

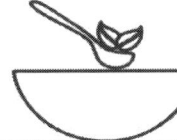 **Lunch**

 **Dinner**

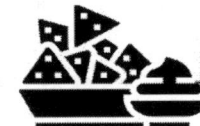 **Snacks**

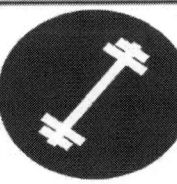 **Workout**

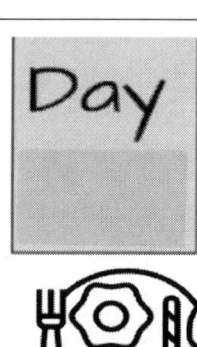 Day

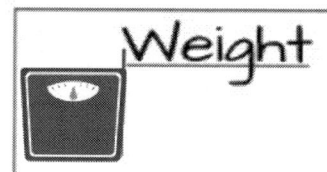 Weight

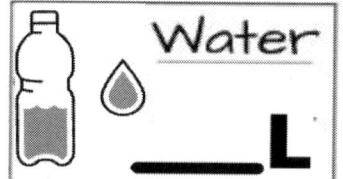 Water ___L

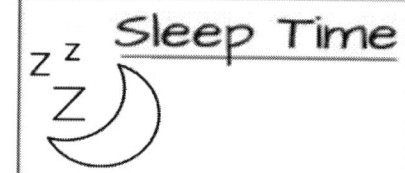 Sleep Time

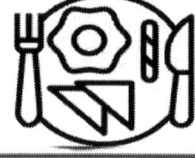 Breakfast

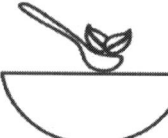 Lunch

 Dinner

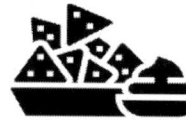 Snacks

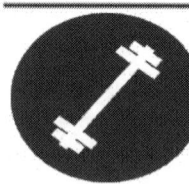 Workout

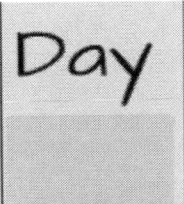 **Day**
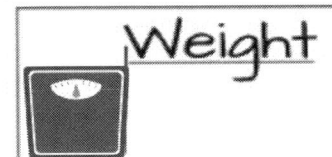 **Weight**
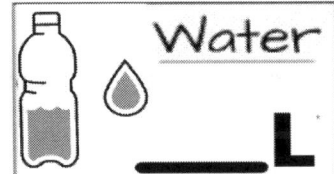 **Water** ___ **L**
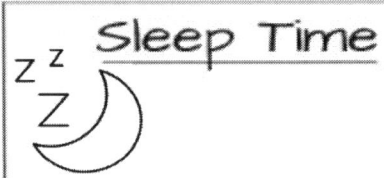 **Sleep Time**

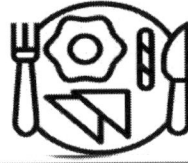 **Breakfast**

 **Lunch**

 **Dinner**

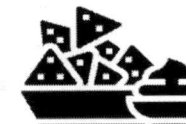 **Snacks**

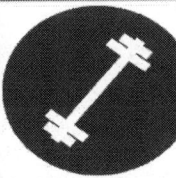 **Workout**

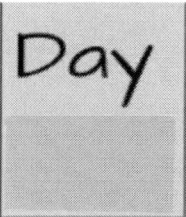 **Day**

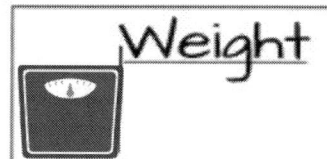 **Weight**

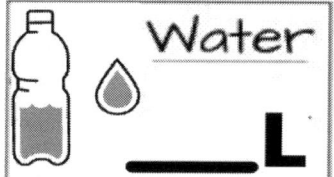 **Water** ___ **L**

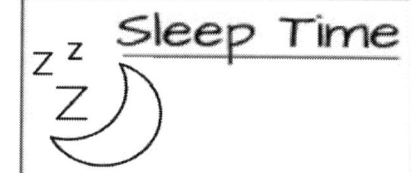 **Sleep Time**

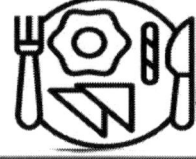 Breakfast

 Lunch

 Dinner

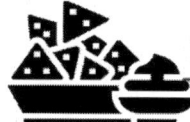 Snacks

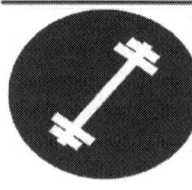 Workout

Made in the USA
Columbia, SC
07 March 2021